Home Health Aide Textbook

Home Care Principles

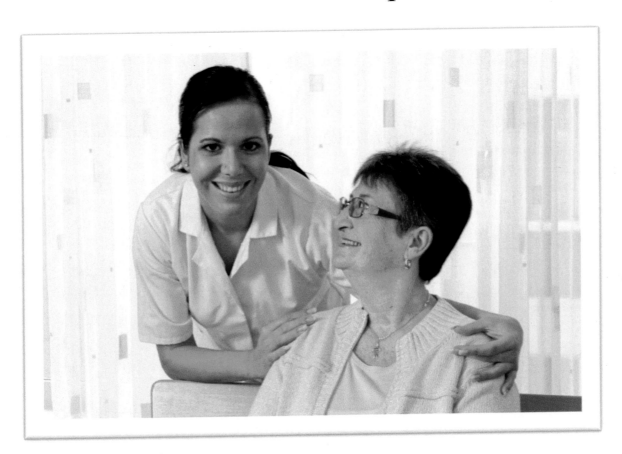

Jane John-Nwankwo CPT, DSD, RN, MSN, PHN

Home Health Aide Textbook

Home Care Principles

ISBN-13: 978-1546656456

ISBN-10: 1546656456

Printed in the United States of America.

Have you bought these books?

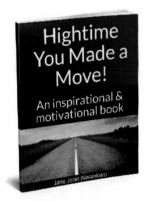
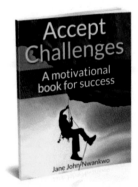
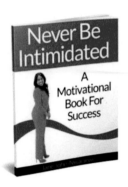

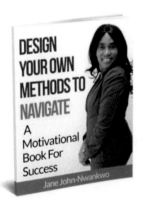
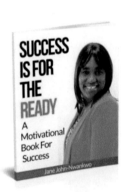
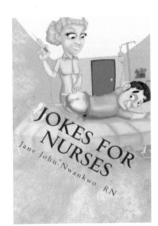

www.janejohn-nwankwo.com

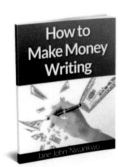
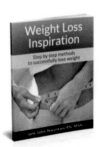
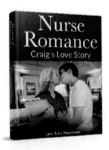
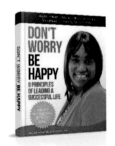

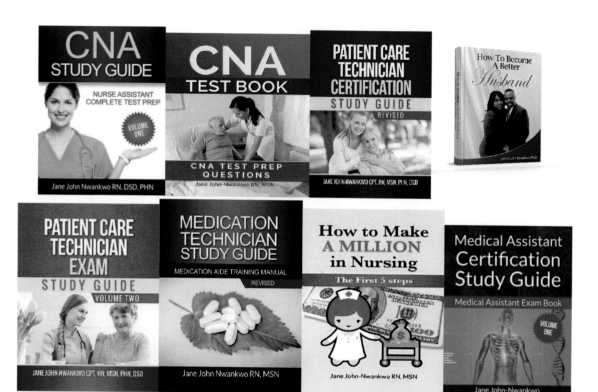

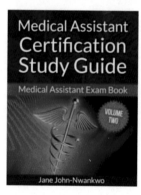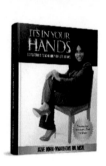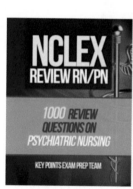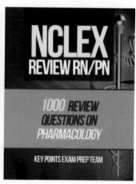

www.janejohn-nwankwo.com

Dedication

To my loving daughter, Jessica Chinyere John-Nwankwo

Table of Contents

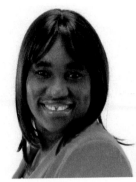

From the author

This book was written out of an inner passion to provide a quality, but concise textbook for Home Health Aides as well as Caregivers. If the reader gains any new knowledge from this book or finds new strength to care for people who require care in their homes, then the purpose of this book would have been achieved.

- Jane John-Nwankwo RN, MSN.

Author, Public speaker,

Educational consultant

support@janejohn-nwankwo.com

www.janejohn-nwankwo.com

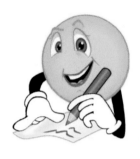

Chapter One

Introduction to the Home Health Agency Role

Outline

1. Introduction

2. State and federal regulations and requirements for HHA certification

3. Purpose and goals of home health care

4. Members of the home health care team

5. Roles and responsibilities of the certified home health aide

6. Common observations and documentation to be done by the HHA

7. Key steps in the communication process and methods of communication

8. Key steps in accommodating communication with clients with hearing or speech disorders.

9. Effective techniques for communication with home health team members

10. Effective communication in learning about clients.

11. Access to community agencies to meet client needs

12. Organizational and time management techniques for a daily work schedule.

13. Conclusion

I. State and Federal Regulations and the requirements for Home Health Aide Certification

In order to become a home health aide, there is no standardized national educational requirement. It depends on which state the HHA is in. While in some states, they don't need any state approved training, other states need them to take state approved classes, pass a competency test and earn a state certification. These classes are usually offered in the community colleges or vocational/technical schools.

Most skill training for HHAs are taught by other healthcare professionals like nurses, and is usually administered during the training period. Usually their training is moduled around the unique needs of home care clients. They also receive orientation on the job.

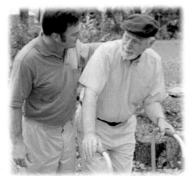 Depending on the level of care needed by the client, the HHA's training could be done from a few hours to a few days. For more complex cases, some employers provide training classes which the aspiring HHA completes before they are given a job.

Most employers would rather hire a Certified Home Health Aide, than an uncertified caregiver. The HHA certification process includes at least 75 hours of training and as much as a 120-hour course in a state like California. It involves the theory section of the training and the skills section. Other requirements may include a background check of candidates before enrolling them to a program due to the professional nature of the job. Sometimes, physical examinations and health screenings like a tuberculosis test may be required to prevent patients from contracting diseases from their caregivers.

II. Purpose and goals of Home Health Care

Home Health Care involves a range of care for a wide variety of patients outside the hospital setting. The services that home health care companies provide can range from nursing care, physical therapy, occupational therapy, speech therapy, etc. from qualified medical professionals to smaller services from home health aides. The care provided could be as simple as assistance in everyday activities such as bathing and eating, to more complex services requiring more specialized professionals. Essentially, the purpose and goal of home care is to provide an adequate level of care in a cost-effective manner while promoting rehabilitation of the patient in a familiar environment like their homes.

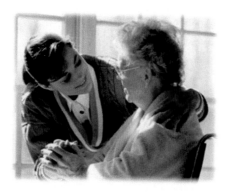

III. Members of the home health care team

Physician - Physicians perform home visits to the patient at regular intervals where they assess the patient in an environment that the patient is more comfortable in. They assess how the patient handles his illness at home. The physician regularly checks and makes adjustments and interventions when necessary. There are two ways in which a physician can function in the home health care setting. One way is by relying on the home health care nurse as the leader, mediator, and coordinator of the group, leaving the physician to be an evaluator of the patient's health to be coordinated with the rest of the team by the nurse.

The other way that the physician can function is to be the one who will lead the team by taking a more active role in patient care. The physician writes prescriptions for the home care client. At the patient's home, the nurses will be able to get a more in-depth assessment of the aspects of the patient's life that is not normally accessible from the hospital setting. In the home, the nurse can look for environmental factors found in the home that could affect the patient's illness, they could see how the patient acts in a more comfortable setting than a hospital, they can assess the patient's compliance with the therapeutic regimen, including diet, exercise, and medications. From these observations, the Registered Nurse can identify some areas that need adjustment in the patient's activities and make interventions to change them for the patient's health. They can also assess the tasks of the health care team and change them to better suit the therapeutic regimen, especially if the Registered Nurse is the one functioning as team leader and coordinator.

Nurse - Most of the care in Home health care is rendered by the nurse. The nurse collaborates with the physician to give the patient the proper care that he needs. They also work with the rest of the personnel in the home health care team to coordinate the services being provided to make sure the patient gets optimal service from each of them to improve the patient's quality of life at home. They perform different nursing interventions adjusted in frequency to suit the patient's needs. During the initial assessment, they also decide which of the other ancillary services are needed by the patient, and this is relayed

to the physician who makes the final decision. The nurse's recommendations influence the interventions ordered by the physician.

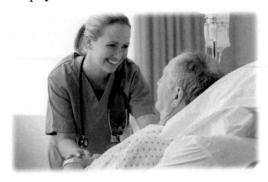

The treatment plans change based on the changes noted by the nurse since they spend the most time with the patient. Because of this, they are the ones in the position to make the comprehensive problems lists and the assessment of care and goal plans. When there are multiple therapies to be done by different members of the home health care team, the nurse schedules the interventions in a way in which they do not overlap so as not to inconvenience the team or stress the patient.

Perhaps one of the most important responsibilities of the nurse is the documentation. They compile all the data about the patient including the treatment plans, prescriptions, and assessments. This serves as a valuable resource to be used by the home health care team, and serves as proof that the team is doing their job. Nurses are also the ones who stay in contact with the whole team, and other community services that could be involved in the patient's care. The nurse updates the rest of the team and allows sharing of information through case conferences.

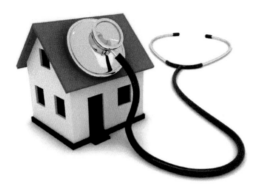

Pharmacist - The role of the pharmacist in the home health care setting is to be responsible for the patient's or caregiver's willingness and ability to be trained to properly administer medications, including the appropriate indications, dose, route, method of administration, and appropriate laboratory tests to monitor the patient's response to the pharmacologic therapy. They use their clinical judgement to know whether the first dose of any drug should be given at the home. It is their job to teach the caregiver about the medications, their effects, adverse effects, any drug interactions, storage and preparation, disposal, special precautions, and general management of drug effects, including emergency procedures. They also make sure that the patient does not run out of medications by checking their stock and by directing them to where they could get medical supplies. The pharmacist works together with the other health care professionals, the patient, and the caregiver in ensuring the appropriate pharmaceutical treatment plan for the patient. They must always be available in case there are any problems, questions, or concerns regarding the pharmacologic treatments. It is important for home health aides to check their state regulations before assisting with medications because most states do not allow HHAs to administer medications.

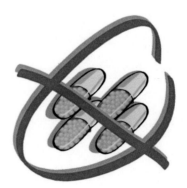

Physical therapist - The physical therapist is needed when the patient has trouble ambulating or has a disability that prevents him from performing everyday tasks.

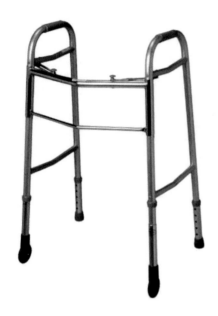

It is their job to assess the patient's disability to determine if the patient needs assistive devices. Once a patient is eligible for an assistive device, the physical therapist is the one to teach the patient its proper use. He also helps the patient increase his mobility and reduce risks of injuries from accidents. He creates the home exercise program to help the patient move around more. During every visit, he assesses the patient's mobility and adjusts the exercises as appropriate to the patient's range of motion, muscle strength, and endurance.

> *The physical therapist is needed when the patient has trouble ambulating or has a disability that prevents him from performing everyday tasks, while the occupational therapist is concerned with how the patient's disease or disability affects their ability to function normally.*

Occupational therapist - The occupational therapist is concerned with how the patient's disease or disability affects their ability to function normally. It is their job to help patients achieve a higher level of independence in everyday tasks such as bathing, dressing, elimination, cooking, eating, and housework. They provide the patient with information about various techniques, equipment, and aids that would allow them to function through their disability. They can help the patient make adjustments to their homes and belongings to improve the patient's functionality; they can teach energy conservation techniques for patients who have low endurance; they are also the ones to teach patients to use specially designed devices to increase their autonomy and functionality. By allowing the patient to do more by himself or herself, their self-esteem increases, and can decrease the need for constant supervision.

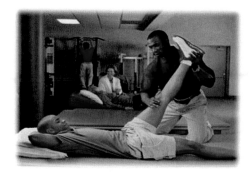

These therapists manipulate the environment of the patient to make it easier for the patient to function, such as widening doors for wheelchairs, grab rails, guide rails, placing objects and switches within arm's reach of the patient, adjusting furniture for easier travel around the house, etc.

Speech therapist - The speech therapist helps patients recover and develop their communication skills for those who have lost the ability to speak normally. They teach compensatory communication mechanisms that uses visual cues and cognitive retraining. They use a wide range of communication aids and technology such as hearing aids, or an electrolarynx; they also teach sign language, and the use of communication boards. As technology for the speech impaired increases, some speech therapist can even teach patients the usage of transcription technology which transcribes spoken words onto a computer screen.

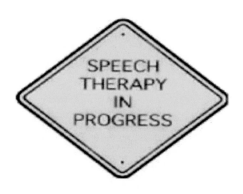

Social worker - The social worker provides emotional and psychological support to the home care team. The social worker is the one with access to community care services when there are conflicts with the treatment plan or if the patient refuses care. When more support is needed in the care of the patient, the social worker assesses the patient with regards to mobility, personal care ability, including an assessment of finances if the patient could afford another professional on the team. They also include the assessments of the rest of the home care team in the making of this decision. The social worker is the link to formal and informal sources of support, whether it comes from social groups, organizations, or help groups. The social worker coordinates, teaches, counsels, assesses, and facilitates ethical decision making issues. They also maintain standards by regular visits and inspections. They are available through a 24-hour emergency call system for the elderly and disabled.

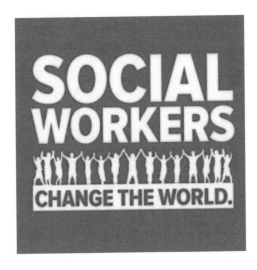

Home Health Aide - The home health aide fulfills the personal care role for the patient. They do the daily tasks of bathing, clothing, positioning, and environmental care of the patient under the supervision of the home care nurse (Kurashi, 2006).

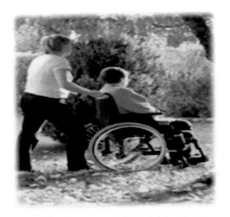

IV. Roles and responsibilities of the certified home health aide.

The certified home health aides fulfill the personal care role for the patient. Home health aides perform under the guidance of the home care nurse, following a written care plan outlining activities and tasks to be done for the patient. This includes the basic tasks of bathing the patient, helping the patient sit upright, position, off, and on to bed, grooming, dental hygiene, basic exercises, and medication. Sometimes, HHAs may help in some household chores such as changing bed linens and keeping the patient's room clean as part of environmental care. Some of these jobs can be done by a trained paid housekeeper. Family members are also candidates for the role of a home health aide (Kurashi, 2006) if they undergo proper training.

V. Common observations and documentation done by the HHA.

According to the Home Health Aide Training Manual by Kay Green (1996), the frequent observations of the HHA include general observations such as weight changes, changes in the ability to perform care, ingestion of alcohol or drugs, fevers, or episodes of weakness; skin observations such as rashes, breaks or tears, changes in color, itching, or bruises; head observations such as headaches, dizziness, fainting spells, and hallucinations;

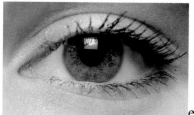 eye observations such as failing eyesight, excessive watering of the eyes, or dryness of the eyes;

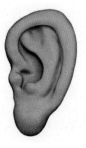 ear observations including hearing ability, tinnitus, or discharge from the ears;

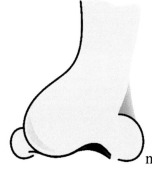 nose and throat observations including congestion, voice changes, nosebleeds, toothaches, patient's dental hygiene, bleeding gums, difficulty swallowing, and halitosis; breast observations such as nipple discharges, lumps, or pains; respiratory system observations including shortness of breath, abnormal breath sounds, coughing, or fluid filled lungs; heart or vascular system observations involving the patient's heart rate, the regularity of his heartbeat, and any chest pains; Stomach and intestinal observations such as the patient's appetite, abdominal discomfort, diarrhea, constipation, vomiting, blood in the stools, and

incontinence; urinary system observations such as the patient's frequency of urination, the color of the urine, incontinence, blood in the urine, the amount of urine, and any pain or difficulty in urination; observations of the patient's genitals such as any abnormal discharges, pain, lesions, and other abnormalities; observations of the patient's musculature such as muscle weakness, neck or back pain, joint pain, cramps, and limitations to movement; Changes in mental/emotional state such as crying, depression, nervousness, and restlessness; and finally neurological system observations such as seizures, numbness, tingling, paralysis, or loss of function. All these observations are to be documented along with the activities done by the HHA during his shift.

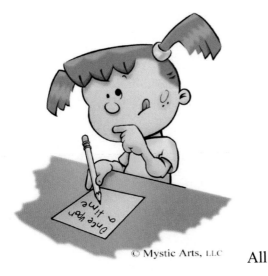

© Mystic Arts, LLC   All these are documented for the benefit of

the patient, the home health care team, and the HHA himself. By documenting these details, the patient's condition can be tracked, and the health care team can identify incremental changes in his condition to adjust the care plan accordingly, while it also protects the HHA since the documentation is a reflection that the HHA is doing his job correctly.

VI. Key steps in the communication process and methods of communication

The key steps in the communication process are Creation, Transmission, Reception, Translation, and Response.

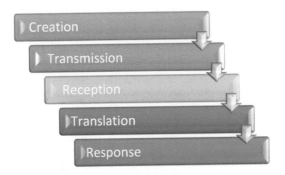

Methods of communication, especially in the home health care setting consist of verbal and non-verbal modes of communication such as written communication (Schreiner, n.d.). Since the HHA has the most contact with the home care client, it is imperative that he reports any changes in the patient condition that is noticed. He should ensure that the data is being transmitted to the right personnel to avoid a breach of patient confidentiality. Clarity in communication is also very essential, avoiding the use of unnecessary abbreviations. E.g. The PT visited the PT. This could mean that the Physical therapist visited the patient, it could also mean that the patient went to the physical therapist office. In any case, there could arise some confusion as to the actual meaning of the documentation. Write in clear simple language that everyone can understand. Avoid cancellations, and if there be a need for cancellations, use only one line across your documentation.

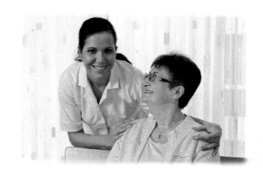

VII. Key steps in accommodating communication with clients with hearing or speech disorders.

It is prudent to keep in mind that this type of communication is difficult, so patience is needed.

The HHA must speak in short, clear sentences; do not use a lot of jargon; use communication tools such as pen and paper, pictures, or sign language if the patient has been taught; If the patient cannot speak, ask yes or no questions instead; use communication aids; consult a speech therapist ("Communicating with patients who have speech/language difficulties," 2009).

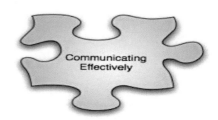

The HHA must speak in a clear manner, loud enough for the patient to hear but at the same time, not shouting. If the client hears better with one hear, stand closer to the ear with a better function. Facing the client with hearing difficulty is often helpful since most of them compensate with lip reading. Never be in a hurry when communicating with clients with hearing or speech disorder; allow them time to finish their sentences and do not assume that you know what they have in mind to say. Encouraging sign language when the client is being trained to recover their speech abilities is not a good rehabilitation technique.

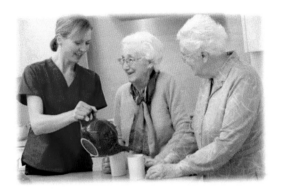

VIII. Effective techniques for communication with home health team members

One of the most effective techniques for communication, and the most important, is the written form of communication of the documentation. This record of everything done by, to, and about the patient is meant to be a non-urgent form of communication between the health team members. It should be regularly updated so that the other team members will be abreast of the patient's current status, view old and current interventions, etc. so that they may be guided accordingly in the care of the patient (Green, 1996).

Another effective technique in communicating with the health team is the case conference. This is a regular meeting of all the members of the team wherein they exchange information and plan for the care of the patient. The verbal and written exchange of this conference results in a treatment plan that covers multiple aspects of the patient's care, making sure that the patient is cared for holistically (Kurashi, 2006).

IX. Effective communication in learning about client.

Effective communication can go a long way to helping learn things about the client. It is important to form a good nurse-patient relationship. To effectively communicate with the client to gain her trust as well as gain information about him/her, the nurse must be prepared with information for the client's questions, maintain eye contact, observe body language, listen closely, pay attention to both verbal and non-verbal cues, avoid medical jargon (phrasing questions in ways the patient will understand), and most of all, be sensitive to the client and choose the right moment to ask questions ("Communication skills", 2007).

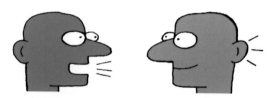

X. Access to community agencies to meet client needs

As stated above, the home care nurse and the social worker both have access to other community agencies and resources. Through the National Association for Home Care and Hospice, here are some of the affiliates and community agencies that could cater to the needs of the client:

Hospice association of America, Private Duty Homecare Association of America, Center for Health Care Law, World Homecare and Hospice Organization,

Pediatric Home Care Association of America, Hospital Home Care Association of America, Proprietary Home Care Association of America, Voluntary Home Care Association of America, Home Medical Equipment Association of America, Psychiatric care services, among others (Kurashi, 2006; "NAHC Affiliates," n.d.)

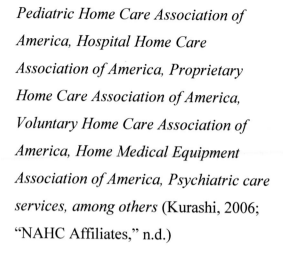

XI. Organizational and time management techniques for a daily work schedule.

According to Wittenberg (2012), there are many ways to save time for a home health aide:

A. Use time management building blocks:

    1. Identify your goals

    2. Review your time utilization

    3. Match time utilization patterns with your goals

    4. Prioritize for better time management

    5. Eliminate time bandits (procrastination, perfectionism, etc.)

B. Use computerized documentation

C. Plan and Manage your schedule ahead of time, including your own self-care time

D. Do the whole job, or one thing at a time.

E. Stay focused

F. Telephone management

G. Stress Management.

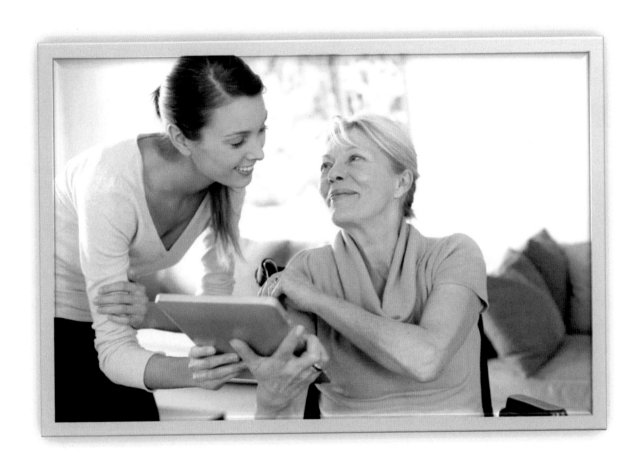

BIBLIOGRAPHY

Wittenberg, S. (2012). Effective Time Management. Retrieved from
   http://nursing.advanceweb.com/Article/Effective-Time-Management-3.aspx

Davila, L. (n.d.). How to become a Home Health Aide. Retrieved from
   http://www.innerbody.com/careers-in-health/how-to-become-a-home-health-
   aide.html

NAHC Affiliates. (2012). Retrieved from http://www.nahc.org/affiliates/home.html

Communication Skills. (2007, Dec 13). *Nursing Times.* Retrieved from
   http://www.nursingtimes.net/nursing-practice/clinical-
   zones/educators/communication-skills-essence-of-care-benchmark/361127.article

Schreiner, E. (n.d.). 5 steps to the communication process in the workplace. Retrieved
   from http://smallbusiness.chron.com/5-steps-communication-process-workplace-
   16735.html

Communication with patients who have speech and language difficulties. (2009).
   Retrieved from http://www.patientprovidercommunication.org/article_2.htm

Green, K. (1996). *Home health aide training manual.* Burlington, MA: Jones & Barlett
   Learning.

Kurashi, N. (2006). Home health care team members. *Middle East Journal of Age and
   Ageing, 3*(1). Retrieved from http://www.me-jaa.com/mejaa6/homehealth.htm

1) ……………..provides assistance to the chronically ill, the elderly, and family caregivers who need relief from the stress of care-giving?

A) Home health Aids

B) Pastors

C) Engineers

D) Surgeons

2) Agencies pay home health aides from payments they receive from the following payers:

A) Insurance companies

B) Health maintenance organizations

C) Medicare

D) All of the above

3) The Centre for Medicare and Medicaid services payment system for home care is called the:

A) Home health prospective payment system

B) Pay per charge

C) Service payment

D) Medical payment

4) Clients who need home care are referred by a doctor to a:

A) Hospital

B) Friend

C) Neighbor

D) Home health agency

5) All home health aides are under supervision of one of the following skilled professionals:

A) An engineer

B) A pastor

C) A registered nurse

D) Native medicine

6) All of the following constitute the team of health professionals except:

A) Home health aides

B) Nurses

C) Doctors

D) Engineers

7) ……………….helps clients learn to compensate for disabilities:

A) A client

B) An occupational therapist

C) Speech language pathologist

D) Registered dietitian

8) A legal term that means someone can be held responsible for harming someone else is referred to as:

A) Assets

B) Liability

C) Action

D) Discipline

9) A particular method, or way, of doing something is called:

A) Orientation

B) A procedure

C) An activity

D) Information

10) A professional relationship with a client includes:

A) Maintaining a negative attitude

B) Not finishing assignments

C) Doing only the tasks assigned

D) None of the above

11) Professionalism means:

A) Having to do with work or a job

B) Your life outside your job

C) Disapproving client's opinion

D) Keeping late to work

12) ....teaches clients and their families about special diets to improve their health and help them manage their illness:

A) A medical social worker

B) A registered dietitian

C) An occupational therapist

D) None of the above

13) A professional relationship with an employer does not include of the following:

A) Always being on time

B) Completing assignments efficiently

C) Maintaining a negative attitude

D) Participating in education programs offered

14) Which of the following depicts the meaning of laws?

A) Laws are rules set by the government

B) Laws tell us what we must do

C) Laws help to ensure order and safety

D) All of the above

15) ....defines the things you are allowed to do and describes how to do them correctly:

A) A plan

B) A liability

C) A procedure

D) A scope of practice

16) Which of the following is not an example of legal and ethical behavior by HHAs?

A) Protecting client's privacy

B) Accepting gifts and tips

C) Being honest at all times

D) Documenting accurately and promptly

17) Clients have the right to:

A) Have access, upon request, to all bills for service the client has received

B) Receive care of the highest quality

C) Refuse services without fear of reprisal

D) All of the above

18) Unexplained injuries including burns, bruises, and bone injuries can be referred to as:

A) Mental abuse

B) Physical abuse

C) Psychological abuse

D) Passive neglect

19) You can help protect your client's rights in which of the following ways:

A) Respect your clients' property

B) Talk or gossip about a client

C) Neglect clients in your planning

D) Enter a client's room without knocking and seeking permission

20) To respect confidentiality means:

A) To tell the a client's best friend about his friend's health condition

B) To keep private things secret

C) To discuss issues about a client with in a family meeting

D) None of the above

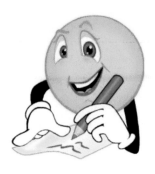

CHAPTER TWO

Medical and social needs of home care clients.

Outline.

1. Introduction

2. Basic physical and emotional needs of clients

3. Recognizing the role of HHA

4. Relating client and family rights to Maslow's hierarchy of needs

5. Culture, lifestyle and life experiences

6. Common reactions to illness/disability

7. Description of basic body functions and changes that should be reported

8. Diseases and disorders common in the healthcare clients

9. Common emotional and spiritual needs

10. Conclusion

1. Introduction.

The home health aide has the role of assisting the client and family in managing the condition of health at the clients home. This chapter will describe the needs of the clients, explain the role of the home health aide and relate the rights of the client and family to Maslow's hierarchy of needs. It will also discuss culture, life style and experiences of clients while identifying common reaction to illness or disability, outline body functions, diseases and disorders and emotional or spiritual needs of patients.

2. Basic physical and emotional needs of clients.

Home health aides help clients who have diverse needs so that they feel comfortable and obtain assistance. They include the elderly, infants, mentally ill, people with physical and developmental disabilities together with people with nutritional needs. Majority of the clients require physical assistance in form of service. They often require to be bathed,

dressed and given a hand to conduct self-grooming. The client needs to be assisted to wash their hands and perform hygienic tasks to control infections. They need someone to support them as they manage pain. The urinal system may be causing incontinence and they will need someone to help them (Harris, 2004, p. 5).

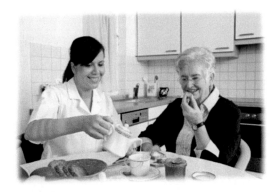

Clients may have nutritional requirements. The home health aide will assist in making the right combination of food and serve them. Those with skin ailments or wounds require help to take care of the skin and the wounds. The home health aide may be required to change the dressing at the right time. It is within the scope of home health aides to change simple dry dressings, however more complex dressing changes would require a licensed nurse. The disabled and the elderly may have musculoskeletal system problem. They will need someone to assist them in mobility. The bedridden will require someone who understands the best position when turning them in bed or moving them to another location. The HHA will give a hand in ambulation and motion. The client will be in need of a safe environment, the home health aide makes the environment safe for the client. They can clean and arrange their house (Eldelman and Madle 2010, p. 22).

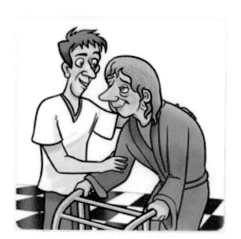

As an important member of the home health team, the HHA is involved in organizing and arranging appointments for the client. Organizing entails arranging the means of transport and accompanying the client to their appointments. At times, she/he assists in doing shopping and cooking appropriate food for the client. They provide company for the client, they keep track of medication taken and appointments with the doctors, they also facilitate the client to participate in certain activities as well as exercise.

The home health aides are required to report on the progress of their client since they work under the supervision of a registered nurse, They can be shown how to check respiration rate and temperature for the purpose of helping in a patient's assessment. They follow the care plan in assisting the client with medication reminders to ensure that the client is complying with the medication regimen. According to Ahroni (1989, p. 77), the client needs to be assisted in lifting and coordinating activities. They need someone to provide physical and emotional company. They call in for help in case of emergencies.

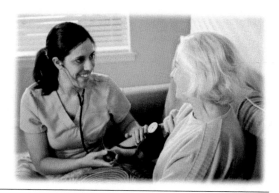

Clients in home health care need emotional support from the home health aide. This can be achieved if they talk to them, share stories, read books, and listen to them. Emotional support is needed by the client as they cope with their condition and situation. The family too, needs emotional support. Families living with the mentally ill patients, disabled and terminally ill need encouragement. The new born can be delicate to handle and people may not be sure how to treat them. The caregivers for the infant may have physical and mental constrains. Emotional support also includes taking the client for recreational activities, walking and accompanying them when they ask.

3. Recognizing the roles of HHA.

Home health aides have the responsibility of ensuring that the client is safe and receives adequate care according to the agreement between the home health agency and the family. Every home care client reserves the same patient's rights as those being cared for in the hospital.

The client or family has the right to be involved when the treatment is being planned. They should be given adequate information on the available services and plans as well as how to gain access or terminate the services. The criteria for eligibility should be clearly outlined. The patient should be made aware of their responsibilities. Services provided should be safe and appropriate. The services should also comply with current medical information. Communication should be efficient to allow the patient know when there are changes in service, schedule and medication.

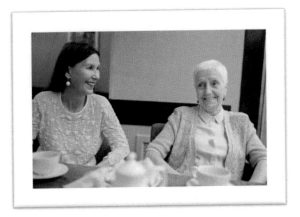

The patient and their family require to be given respect and privacy by the home health aide. The medical information should be kept confidential. The client and their family should not be exploited, mistreated or made uncomfortable. The home health aide can develop a disciplined way of dealing with the patient. For instance, they should avoid yelling, smoking, or ignoring the patient. The patient should be informed about changes in payment when payment is adjusted. The information should be given in advance before changes are made.

Another role of the home health aide is giving quality healthcare. They should respond to the patient's concerns appropriately and in time. Services should be of good quality and should be available when required. Quality of health care is informed by healthcare standards and regulations.

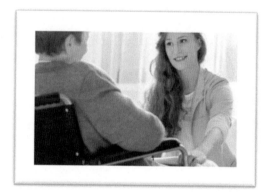

In case the patient's status is not improving the home health aide should ensure that they report the progress of the client to the appropriate institution in time. They should be prepared to support and assist the client in the case of emergency. They should inform the patient and family on the necessary procedure and what has caused the action. It is the home health aide duty to ensure they make arrangement together with the patient or family to have the appropriate resources needed. When any service is beyond the scope of the HHA, the registered nurse, usually called the case manager should be informed.

In the case of absenteeism, the home health aide should inform the home health agency, patient or family in advance. They should be cleared if they have terminated the services, are on leave or will come after some time. The home health aide should cooperate and partner with the client and family to provide care. They should not be discriminatory about their religion, culture, gender or race. Being in constant contact with patient gives them the opportunity to establish a relationship with the client to create a good avenue for bringing in emotional and physical support.

Professionalism is required of the home health aide

4. Relating client and family rights to Maslow's hierarchy of needs.

Maslow's hierarchy of needs is an analysis of human needs. Maslow proposes that people chase the fundamental needs first and proceed to successive needs to form a hierarchy (Maslow, 1970, p. 37). When self-actualization needs are met, the person is believed to have acquired growth. Satisfaction of needs is attained as level in hierarchy is accomplished.

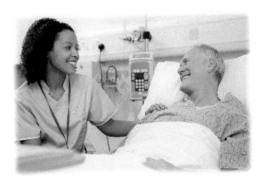

Therefore, the bottom level in the hierarchy contains the most important needs, while the highest level contains the less important needs. The first level at the bottom of the hierarchy is the physiological level. It entails needs such as water, food, rest, sleep and sex. The client and their family in home care are entitled to the basic needs related to homeostasis. The client, whether elderly, disabled, convalescent or infant should be entitled to access the required food, clean water, and get assisted incase their condition requires oxygen administration. Those are basic requirements for sustenance of life.

The second level from the bottom of the hierarchy is the safety level. The safety needs include: health, environmental safety, availability of resources and employment. The clients and their families have the right to enjoy good health. They have a right to secure environment and not to be exposed to danger. The availability of resources enhances the security of the client and their family. Clients have a need to restore their health and live without ailments. In case they are infants and disabled, they need to

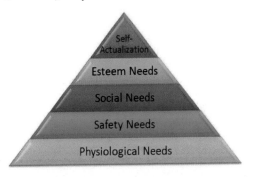

be prevented from exposure that could lead to poor health, injuries, sickness or harm. The family and client need medication and a safe environment where they can be comfortable and secure. They need to be assured that procedures and services offered when receiving home health care are safe.

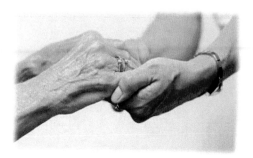

The third level from the bottom of hierarchy is the belonging level. People have a desire to feel that they have friends, feel loved and belong to a family. The family of the client should be encouraged to give support to the client. Emotional support from the home health aide will facilitate the feeling of belonging to the client and the family. The client and the family have a right to express and to be shown love. Every human being is entitled to be treated with respect and dignity. Politeness should be exercised when dealing with the client and family.

The fourth level is called self-esteem. Esteem needs include respect, accomplishment, self-esteem and confidence. The client and the family

need to experience respect from the home health care team. The home health aide must exercise reverence as they give service. Insult, disrespect and lack of kindness could be considered a violation of their rights. When respect is not granted the patient may lack confidence and loose self-esteem. Maintaining self-esteem will provide a platform for giving emotional support. Esteem is one of the important needs when it comes to mental, physical, social and emotional needs.

The topmost level is self-actualization. The needs are reflected on morality, ability to make decisions and renewal of mind. Morality and ethical considerations of the client and family must be considered.

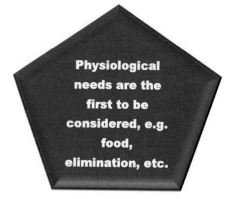

There are professional ethics and laws that are provided for the home health care which must be observed. The home health aide will provide all the information concerning the treatment plan, condition of the client's health, and notify them when there is change in schedule, treatment or payment. The home health aide will ensure that they do not withhold important information on emergency or change in health that requires immediate attention.

5. Culture, lifestyle and life experiences.

Understanding the culture, experience and lifestyle of the client and family will enable the home health aide learn the preferences and attitudes when giving their service. Belonging to a specific community, religion, or any group of people is not a good way of establishing the reasons for the client and their family's behavior. Decision making should be based on their choices and attitude.

Culture, lifestyle and life experience dictates what values the client and the family has. It is necessary to observe the relationship of the client and their family. Cultural values could affect choices of health in different patients. For instance, some ailments or disability may be associated with negative meaning. People vary in experience because they grow up and live in diverse regions. Understanding their lifestyle could give ideas if their ailment could have been caused by their choice of lifestyle. Cultural values could give ideas on how to treat an elderly person.

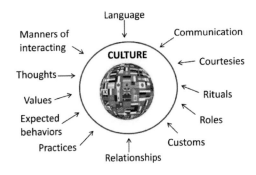

Furthermore, it will give information on the kind of language to be used. This could bring in new ideas like introducing an interpreter. It is not advisable to touch every object one sees in a client's home as some objects may hold sacred significance. When a HHA is assigned to a client, it is the professional duty of the HHA to familiarize themselves with the family. For example, ask how the client prefers to be addressed. For some individuals, addressing them by their first name or other pet names like *honey* or *sweetie* may be insultive.

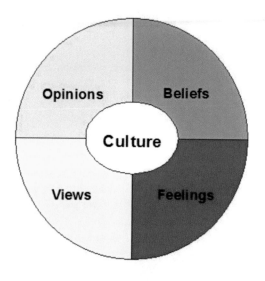

Wernig and Sorrentine (1989, p. 81) note that people value culture and respect it. Culture is the sum total of the way of life of an individual or a group of people. The home health aide should show respect to the client's culture and desist from *ethnocentrism* which means thinking that one's culture is superior to another person's culture. The more respect and cultural diversity observed, the more comfortable the client and their family will be with the agency. Failure to recognize their cultural values and beliefs could lead to mistrust. Obviously, this can be avoided. The home health

aide can engage into a relationship with the client and the family to find out what their feelings are and if they are exercising any fear about the client's condition. Treating a person with dignity and giving quality care could be seen as a significant way of giving value to the client. Identifying cultural prejudices is an effective way of becoming culturally aware. When one pays attention to their beliefs and cultural practices, they choose to adjust their behavior to treat them right. It is very easy to say to oneself "I respect other people's culture, this section of the book is not for me". But take time to ask your self the following questions:

1. How do I feel when someone who has a different accent speaks to me?

2. Do I feel my food is superior when I perceive the odor of foods from other cultures?

3. Do other people's dressing make me uncomfortable?

4. Do I feel people do not know what they believe just because they do not believe in my own God?

Depending on an individual's culture, lifestyle and experience, the home health aide should assess beliefs about sickness and death. They contribute to understanding attitude towards health, attitude on the service of the home health aide, alternative ways of gaining health, religious beliefs, family influence, communication and the client's opinion about their health.

Ethnocentrism is the feeling that one's culture is

Because of lifestyle and life experience, the client and family may have perceptions about medical care and home healthcare aides.. They may have negative or positive experience with the healthcare system. Negative experience could cause a client who is elderly or disabled refuse to cooperate. One can also establish the decision making of the family.

There are cases where the family male head makes decision, while in other families members discuss and give a common answer.

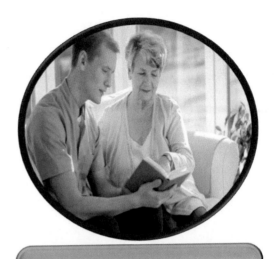

Culture is the way of life of the people

The client may be able to give their decisions and they should be considered. Matters of religion can play a major role in the way the client and family perceives illness. While some may reject some treatment and choose other alternatives, others believe in supernatural power of healing. Depending on experience and culture, clients and family will have diverse response to the home health care. In order to explain the effect of culture on illness, let me discuss a bit about the Igbo culture in Nigeria, West Africa.

THE IGBO CULTURE

The Igbo people usually called 'Ibo' by non-Igbos are situated in the southeast region of Nigeria in West Africa. The area is divided by the Niger River into two unequal sections – the eastern region which is the larger part, and the Midwestern region. The global health case study states that 'According to Nigeria's National Census (1991), the Igbo cultural group accounted for 25 million of the 88.9 million people in the country'.

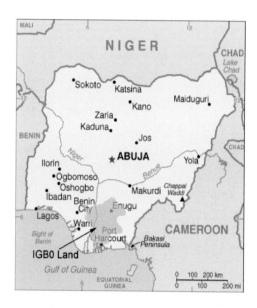

The population reference bureau updates that Nigerian population had increased to 140 million in 2006, and the southern states of which the Igbos constitute a large part of accounted for 65 million. The Igbos speak the Igbo language, and they have two major religions : Christianity and traditional religion. Christianity is the belief in Jesus as the son of God, and Lord, while their traditional religion is the worship of idols, believing that many of the idols are small gods that point to 'Chukwu' meaning the big God. The Igbos are known to value education, hence in present day Igbo culture, the minimum education one would have is the high school certificate. Actually high school graduates are considered illiterates.

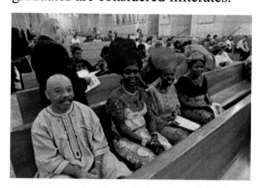

Their staple food is 'Garri' which is processed from cassava. It could be drunk as a cereal, or baked into cakes. But the most common way of eating it is to make it as a dough, and eat it with different kinds of soups. Mostly vegetable packed soups. Other staple foods are Rice and Yam, to name a few.

The cultural practices of the Igbos include: 'The new yam festival' which is usually celebrated around October of every year when the new yam is harvested; 'Igba Nkwu Nwanyi' meaning pouring wine for the bride. This is the name given to their costly marriage ceremony, where the groom has to spent the savings of a long

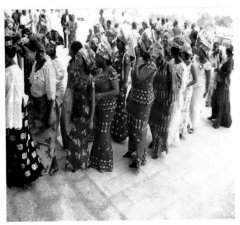

period to get married. This usually contributes to the longevity of the Igbo marriages, if unfaithfulness is noted or other conflicts, and the lady decides to go home to her parents, another ceremony is performed.

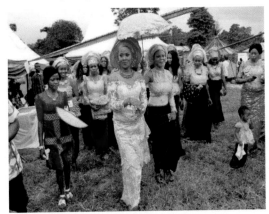

This practice has helped couples to

resolve their differences on time before it gets out hand. Of course there are several other practices which the scope of this book will constrain me to write.

The health beliefs of this ethnic group in relation to health and illness include the following:

- That most illnesses are caused by one's enemies who submitted their names to evil sprits.
- That some illnesses are a reward of one's evil doing in the past.
- That evil spirits could be appeased to cure mysterious illnesses.
- That health is a gift from God (Chukwu) and should be maintained by good food, so the eating of fruits and vegetables is usually the norm, as these vegetables are mostly grown from family gardens and are not bought in the market. Even if they are bought, they are very affordable.
- That husbands should stick to their wives sexually to prevent 'Nsi Nwanyi' meaning myserious illness gotten from women. This is the common name for sexually transmitted diseases.
- The use of local herbs to cure illnesses which have been proven to be effective over the ages.

The specific health and illness needs of the Igbo people include:

● Lack of portable drinking water: Water is usually bought from some rich people that installed bore-hole systems. The public tap water which is the main source of water supply is not usually maintained by the government because of misappropriation of funds. This water problem is usually worse during the dry season, because during the rainy season. The source of water supply is usually Rainfall.

● Most families are low income earners and the staple foods which are garri, yam and rice are usually costly. So under nourishment is usually a problem which could be solved by the assisted nutritional services like food stamps or free food programs.

● The main disease or illness suffered by this group is Malaria. But there have been many resources and curative measures available, so mortality from malaria is almost a thing of the past.

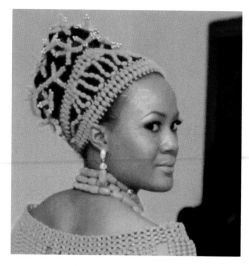

● According to a global health case study, 'Agriculture is a heritage occupation and remains quite traditional with small sized farms, and rain-fed crop production. All crops cultivated are used as food. Nonetheless, both protein-energy and micronutrient deficiencies are a public health problem'.

● Over-crowding is a major problem as people are over-crowded in cars, schools, and living places. This usually aids in the transmission of infectious diseases easily.

● Majority of the Igbo people suffer from and die from stroke since healthcare is not affordable for early diagnoses of the illness. And to make it worse, when somebody slumps on the way in a real village setting, no help is called for as it is believed that the evil spirits tormenting the individual would start tormenting the helper. This is recently improving with the continuous health education on heart attacks, and strokes.

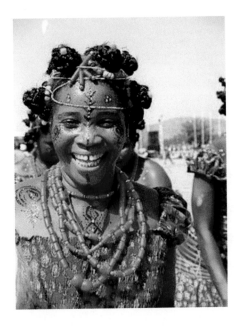

Road traffic accidents (RTA) is one of the major causes of death in this area, because of lack of proper driving regulations. A health education research supports this by stating that 'Data taken from admissions records to the hospital and private clinics (the three facilities which treat accidents) show a similar dominance of RTAs. All entries relating to unintentional injuries were extracted for 1 year, from March 1993 to March 1994. Ninety-nine entries were recorded, of which 63 were injuries caused by

RTAs'.

Their ways of meeting healthcare needs include the following:

- Since there is no health insurance, and health delivery is usually based on availability of cash payment by the patient, people usually go to the hospital when they are really sick. This aids in a high rate of mortality level because in some cases, the illnesses are at their end stage.

- Thanks to the government of the Igbo people that both over the counter drugs and prescriptions drugs can be gotten over the counter even with no prescription. And medications are sold relatively cheap, far cheaper than that what hey are sold here in the United States. Hence antibiotics, anti-malarial drugs, and most common diseases can be easily bought, and one follows the dosage on the drugs. If not for this, millions of people would have died because they could not afford hospital bills.

Home Health Aides must embrace Cultural diversity

- Many deliveries are done by experienced traditional midwives or people that have have some background in healthcare, and this is done either in their homes, or in their some small private clinics. This reduces the cost of child birth, and pregnant mothers are usually referred to the hospitals if their pregnancy is complicated. The negative effect is that many babies are lost, and some mothers do not make it to the hospital.

- Apart from traditional midwives helping in deliveries, they also help in circumcision of males. There are also herbalists that are known and proven to use herbs to cure illnesses.

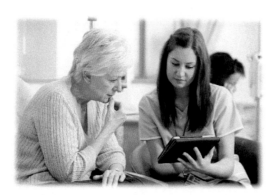

- Some herbs like 'Akum, shut up!' are grown by most people in their back yard. 'Akum' means malaria, shut up is an English language. This herb is very

bitter, but when soaked in water and drunk, cures malaria. Keep in mind that malaria is the commonest illness in this culture, although the fatality has greatly reduced because of availability of its cure in various ways.

Some areas of conflict between cultural practices and the healthcare delivery system include the following:

- The strong belief that one's illness is caused by one's enemies prevents people from seeking healthcare delivery, because it is believed to be useless in such cases. Many people die because of this belief.

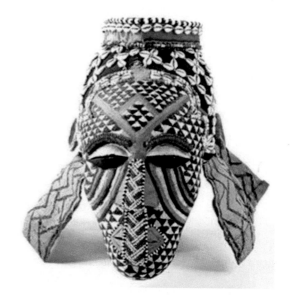

- The smuggling in of herbal

preparations into the hospitals usually affects real assessment of the success of the treatment plan. Usually nurses make it a routine to search patients' surroundings to make sure that there are no hidden preparations.

- Some people do not want to be blamed for not going to the hospital, so they go, but cheek their medications, and throw them away when the nurse leaves the room, fake recovery after a few two or three days from admission, and go home. This could either be from believing in a non-scientific origin of the illness, or other personal beliefs.

- It is usually a thing of pride to have a non-eventful pregnancy, which is crowned by a vaginal delivery of the baby. Hence many women try everything they can to have vaginal delivery to maintain their ego, as people who have not gone through normal delivery and gone through the pains of childbirth are not 'real women'. Some end up losing their babies or their lives in the process of being 'real women'. The home health aide should practice attentive listening to understand why the client believes in what they hold fast.

Personal biases should be relegated to the side.

6. Common reactions to illness/disability.

It is important for the home health aide student to be prepared in dealing with the reaction of the client and family on their condition or illness. The elderly, convalescent, disabled and infants may not be able to perform certain duties. Additionally, their condition may not allow them to generate income. This means that they are dependent on others for service and financial support. If the financial burden is very high on the family, family constraints can occur. Some families have insurance and get the relief.

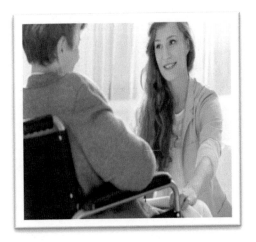

Some family members may not be willing to give service, for fear of contracting the disease or other reasons like dedication to job or just not being able to cope with the stress of a loved one that is dependent. The burden of taking care of the client may be left to one person. As the family gives support to the client, they develop emotional, psychological and physical needs. They may end up with limited time to take care for themselves.

The challenge emerging from the home health care can cause depression to the patient and family. Demands for more resources and time can be tiring. Moreover, taking care of the patient could be very demanding and cause stress. If the patient does not show any improvement after the services of the home health agency have been employed, anxiety may crop in for lack of progress. They may live in worry; lose self-esteem and start experiencing moments of grief because of client's condition. If stress on the part of the client and their family is not managed well they could end up in destructive behaviors. The client may attempt to withhold from treatment, the family may ignore their responsibility and become hostile or on the other extreme, become over-protective. Home health environment where working relations are constrained and the family is fully or partially withdrawn from giving support may become stressed. Good relationship between a client and their family facilitate creating a complimentary environment for home care.

Assessing the needs of the client and that of the family will inform the plan when giving service. The home health aide should evaluate the most important and the less significant needs and give priority according to the needs. It is necessary to give the family and the client relevant information that can help them cope with the situation. Getting them to increase their knowledge about the circumstances will give them a reason for negative reactions. Family members who feel overburdened by the demands of the resources could seek alternatives such as insurance. They can be referred to a program that educates and provides support for people with similar health needs.

In the case where one of the family members is overburdened with responsibilities, arrangements can be made to reduce the burden. The family can request support from other family members to get economic relief resulting from the conditions of the client. There is need to treat depression and stress to facilitate good health. Training on how to deal with the special need of the client can be given. Engaging in a program will facilitate an opportunity for the family and client to share with others and reduce the chances of getting stressed (Doenges et al, 2010, p. 67).

7. **Description of basic body functions and changes that should be reported.**

Basic body functions can be explained by understanding the functions of the organs of the body. The integumentary system is responsible for normalizing temperature of the body, generate hormones and support the sensory organs. Skeletal system facilitates body movements, stores blood cells and minerals. Muscular organs give the body posture, warmth and enables movement. The nervous system enables communication and control between the surrounding and the body. Endocrine

body functions include generation and distribution of hormones to the blood. Circulatory system distributes immunity and required substances to different parts of the body. The lymphatic system facilitates transportation of fluids in the body.

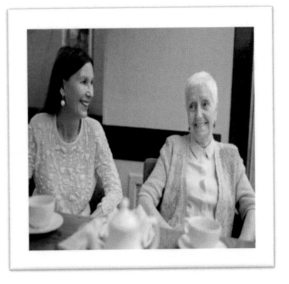

The respiratory system basic function is to excrete carbon dioxide and inhale oxygen. The digestion enables the body transform food into nutrients and excretes the unwanted waste from the body. Urinary organs remove waste, and create a balance between acid and electrolytes with water. Reproductive organs are responsible for generating sex cells and allowing transfer as well as fertilization to produce new offspring.

The home health aide should ensure that they report any changes that threaten the life of the client. This may include persistent respiratory difficulties, frequent falls and reduced level of consciousness that cannot be explained. They should report when the blood sugar is very high despite medication. Similarly, very high blood pressure or very low blood pressure. Drug reactions must also be reported for the physician to make adjustments. The home health aide should make it a routine to report to the home health care agency the client's progress (Birchenall, 2012, p. 61).

8. Diseases and disorders common in the healthcare clients.

There are diseases and disorders that HHAs should be aware of because they are common in home health care. The elderly people complain of Dementia. Dementia is characterized by impaired cognition and loss of memory. The elderly demonstrates neurological disorders. Neurological disorders signs can include pain in the muscle especially when making movement. The elderly may suffer from incontinence. Symptoms of incontinence are loss of control of bladder.

Another common disease in the elderly is cardiovascular disease. Some may experience a heart attack, cardiac arrest or high blood pressure. The Arthritis is another disease common in home care. Signs of arthritis include pain in the ankle, knee, feet, wrist, hip, hands, back, spine, neck and shoulder. Elderly have challenges with their vision and earring. Their vision becomes blurred and they may require one to talk aloud enough so that they can hear (Shouting is avoided). The vision problems could have been caused by glaucoma or muscular degeneration. Some elderly clients have diabetes. Signs and symptoms include blood glucose that is high, sweating and blurred visions. Some have sleeping disorders.

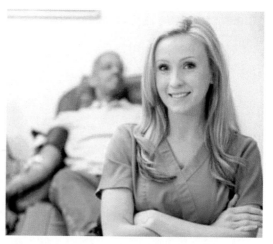

The elderly may have osteoporosis.

Osteoporosis makes bones break easily and takes a long time to heal, and cause injuries and sprains. Other clients may have lung disease, which causes them to breath with difficulty. Skin disorders are common in home health care. Skin disorder signs include irritation of the skin, rashes and sensitive skin (Sommers, 2010, p. 25).

Cancer is another disease prevalent in home care. Cancer is an abnormal proliferation of cells can affect any part of the body. In any cancerous cell, there is growth without control. There are various forms of cancer, others are gender based. The client could suffer from cognitive disorders. It could be in for of delirium syndrome. The symptoms include disturbed conscience, disorganized thoughts and agitation.

9. Common emotional and spiritual needs.

A terminally ill client together with their family has different emotional and spiritual needs. They have different abilities to cope with the situation. While some may be in denial, others may have accepted reality. Majority of the terminally ill patient go through the grieving process. They first deny the news and isolate themselves. They experience anger and strong emotions of despair. They quickly realize the reality and begin to bargain on the life in their thoughts. They then enter into a depression. Finally, they accept the reality and begin to give their best in the remaining days. The home health aide understands that the family undergoes Kubler-Ross stages of grief which has the acronym: DABDA. D-Denial, A-Anger, B-Bargaining, D-Depression, A-Acceptance.

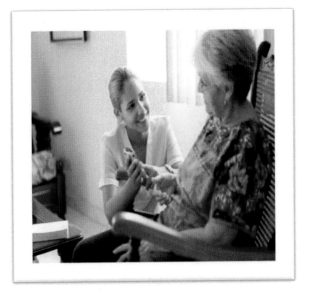

The terminally ill and the family agonize and feel pain for the anticipated loss. The terminally ill experiences pain from the illness. They have feelings of helplessness for not being able to accomplish all they wanted in life. The patient may go into depression because they are not able to meet their responsibilities. The family members become depressed after seeing that they cannot restore the health of their loved one (Birchenall and Streight, 2003, p. 11).

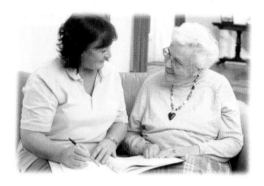

The interventions for emotions include allowing the patient and the family talk to a therapist or counselor about their experience. One can facilitate and organize for the family to spend a lot of time with each other. They can be encouraged to share their thoughts and feelings. In their discussion they can be helped to deal with anxiety and fear. This can be done by showing them how to relax. They can exercise breathing exercise. Their concerns on medication and treatment for comfort should be conversed. Allowing the client time to express their feelings is very important. Bottled emotions do not help with

coping. Venting emotions helps to relax the muscles and helps client to explore ways that can serve as coping strategies.

Spiritual support involves inviting the client's religious leader for spiritual guidance. The client and family can be encouraged to get the support from their clergy. Interacting with the clergy will create avenues for asking questions and obtaining answers about spiritual matters. The religious leader can provide spiritual support which is effective in dealing with anxiety (Stanworth, 2003, p. 30).

10. Conclusion.

The client needs someone to help them bath, dress do self-grooming, control infections, take medication, get help in mobility, manage pain, safe environment and get help with cleaning. They need company and encouragement as emotional support. The home health aide should follow the care plan in providing service. The client and family, just like every other individual follow Maslow's hierarchy of needs which include the physiological, safety, belonging, esteem and self-actualization needs. Culture, lifestyle and experience of client and family motivate their decision making and perception about the condition of the client. Illnesses and disability cause financial constraints and need for service. Support helps the client and family deal with constraints. Changes such as unconsciousness, persistent high blood sugar and persistent difficulty in breathing should be reported. Many clients in home care have Dementia, neurological disorders, incontinence, cardiovascular disease, arthritis, poor vision, hearing difficulties, diabetes, osteoporosis, sleeping disorders, cancer and cognitive disorders. The client and family need encouragement when the patient is terminally ill. They can be given support by their religious leaders.

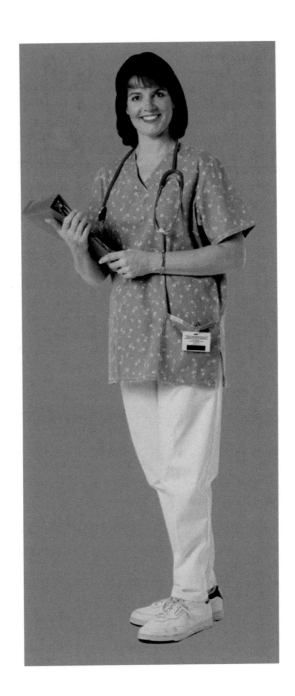

BIBLIOGRAPHY

Ahroni, J. H. (1989). A description of the health needs of the elderly home care patients with chronic illness. *Home Health Care Service Quarterly,* 10, 3, 77-92.

Birchenall, J. M. (2012). Mosby's Textbook for the Home Aide. New Jersey: Mosby.

Birchenall, J. M., and Streight, E. (2003) Mosby's Textbook for the Homecare aide, 2nd edition, New Jersey: Mosby.

Doenges, M., Moorhouse,M., and Murr, A. (2010) Nurse's Pocket Guide: Diagnoses, Prioritized Interventions and Rationales. Philadelphia: F.A. Davis Company.

Eldelman, C. L., and Madle, C. L. (2010). Health promotion throughout the Life span, seventh edition. New Jersey: Mosby.

Harris, M. D. (2004). Handbook of Home Health Care Administration. London: Jones & Bartlett Publishers.

Maslow, A. H. (1970). Motivation and personality, 2nd edition., New York: Harper and Row.

Sommers, M. (2010) Diseases and Disorders: A Nursing Therapeutics Manual. Philadelphia: F.A. Davis Company.

Stanworth, R. (2003) Recognizing Spiritual Needs in People who are Dying. Oxford: OUP Oxford.

Wernig, J. K., and Sorrentine, S. A. (1989). Homemaker- Home Health Aide. *Journal of Health Occupation and Education,* 5, 1, 81-82.

SAMPLE HOME HEALTH AIDE QUESTIONS

21) ………………..is the process of exchanging information with others:

   A) Looking

   B) Recreation

   C) Communication

   D) Interpretation

22) Always report combative behaviors of clients to your:

   A) Parents

   B) Client's friend

   C) Friend

   D) Supervisor

23) All of the following are some barriers to communication, except:

   A) Client hears and understands you clearly

   B) Client is difficult to understand

   C) Asking why

   D) Client speaking in a different language

24) Which of the following questions would you ask a client for adequate clarifications?

   A) Did you sleep last night?

   B) Did he rape you?

   C) Tell me about your sleep last night

   D) Is exercise good?

25) Reasons for documentation include:

   A) It guarantees clear and complete communication

   B) It provides up-to-date record of the status of a client

   C) Documentation protects you and the employer from liability

   D) All of the above

26) File an incident report when one of the following incidents occurs:

   A) You client performs an exercise

   B) Your client falls

   C) When a patient is safe

   D) When a client lies on the right side of the body

27) The process of removing pathogens or state of being free from pathogens is referred to as:

   A) Medical asepsis

   B) Plasmodiasis

   C) Sepsis

   D) Toxoplasmosis

28) …………..is where the pathogen lives and grows:

   A) House

   B) Ecosystem

C) Landscape

D) Reservoir

29) An uninfected person who could get sick or infected is referred to as a:

A) Portal of entry

B) Causative agent

C) Susceptible host

D) Sepsis

30) If blood or body fluid spills on fabrics such as carpets and clothes:

A) Use alcohol to clean it

B) Use commercial disinfectants to clean it

C) Clean with bleach

D) None of the above

31) ………………..is a federal government agency that issues information to protect the health of individuals and communities:

A) Health firm

B) World health organization

C) The centre for disease control and prevention

D) Individual co-operations

32) One of the following is not included as one of the measures of standard precautions:

A) Clean a client's blood without wearing gloves

B) Wash your hands before putting on gloves

C) Wear gloves if you may come in contact with body fluids

D) Wear a disposable gown that is resistant to body fluid

33)………………..refers to washing hands with water and soap or other detergents that contain an antiseptic agent:

A) Hand antisepsis

B) Hand rinsing

C) Protocols

D) None of the above

34) Equipment that helps protect employees from serious injuries or illnesses resulting from contact with workplace hazards is called:

A) Personal protective equipment

B) Standard precaution

C) Hospital policy

D) Health machineries

35) Personal protective equipment includes the following, except one:

A) Masks

B) Goggles

C) Gowns

D) Needles

36) One of the following is not an airborne disease:

A) Measles

B) Tuberculosis

C) Boil

D) Chickenpox

37) Droplets can be created by:

A) Coughing

B) Sneezing

C) Laughing

D) All of the above

38) An example of a droplet disease is the:

A) Rash

B) Scabies

C) Mumps

D) Constipation

39) MRSA stands for:

A) Menstrual reluctant stage of Action

B) Men Rehabilitation system activities

C) Methicillin-resistant staphylococcus aureas

D) None of the above

40) Droplet precautions include:

A) Wearing a face mask during care

B) Restricting visits from uninfected people

C) An infected client covering his nose and mouth with a tissue when sneezing

D) All of the above

41) The way the parts of the body works together whenever you move is referred to as:

A) Body mechanics

B) Movement

C) Body structure

D) Matrix

42) When you stand, your weight is centered in:

A) Elbows

B) Your arms

C) Your pelvis

D) Fibula

43) Disorientation means confusion about:

A) Person

B) Place

C) Time

D) All of the above

44) Burns can be caused by one of the following:

A) Cold water

B) Hand shaking

C) Dry heat

D) Waxing floors

45) Employee's responsibilities for infection control include the following:

A) Follow standard precautions

B) Take advantage of the free hepatitis B vaccination

C) Immediately report any exposure you have to infection, or blood

D) All of the above

46) One of the following is not a guideline to guide against fire:

A) Stay in or near the kitchen when anything is cooking

B) Discourage careless smoking and smoking in bed

C) Turn on heaters when no one is home

D) Do not leave dryer on when you leave the house

47) To ensure travel safety:

A) Avoid planning your route

B) Use turn signals

C) Encourage distractions from friends

D) Drive without seat belt

48) Factors that raise the risk for falls include:

A) Clutter

B) Slippery floors

C) Poor lighting

D) All of the above

49) …………..is emergency care given immediately to an injured person?

A) Exercise

B) Head stretching

C) 9111

D) First aid

50) The first signs of insulin reaction include one of the following:

A) Pneumonia

B) Heart failure

C) Constipation

D) Nervousness

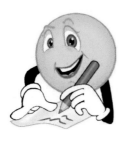 # CHAPTER THREE

Personal Care Services by the Home Health Aide

Outline

1. Introduction
2. Steps and guidelines for common personal care
3. Importance of improvising equipment and adapting care activities in the home
4. Personal care delivery at home
5. Examples of equipment that can be used to provide care
6. Benefits of self-care in promoting wellness
7. Key principles of body mechanics
8. How to adapt body mechanics in the home
9. Adaptations that can be made in the home for ambulation and positioning
10. The purpose of passive and active range motion exercise
11. High risk factors for skin breakdown and methods of prevention
12. Stages of pressure ulcers/decubitus ulcers and report observation
13. Types of ostomies and how to empty and change the pouch
14. Emergencies in the home and critical steps to follow
15. The chain of infection to the home care setting
16. Infection control measures to use in the home care setting
17. Role and responsibilities of the HHA in assisting the client to self-administer medications
18. Conclusion

Personal Care Services by the Home Health Aide

1. Introduction.

Personal care is important in the management of home care clients. Personal care enables the client to feel comfortable and prevent other illnesses. This chapter will discuss personal care, equipment needed and taking care of the skin. It will also talk about infection and the role of home health aide in self-administered medications.

2. Steps and guidelines for common personal care.

The client in need of home healthcare usually requires assistance in personal care. The home health aide should have skills such as bed bath, tub bathing and shower bathing. They should be very familiar with the guidelines of transferring or lifting the client when they want to change position. Personal care skills will also include lifting the patient from the floor. The personal care skills are necessary because the client may not be able to move independently. Their mobility can be limited because they suffered from a stroke that may have caused brain damage, body weakness or caused them to have unusual posture. Correct steps in personal care eases positioning and transfer as well as, maintains comfort for the client. The steps and guidelines in personal care assist in fostering safety when moving the client. The client and the home health aide reduce the chances of injury when conducting personal care. (Birchenall 2012, p. 33)

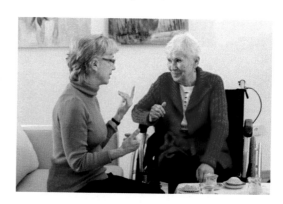

A bed bath is refreshing, allows skin inspection and allows change of beddings. A bed bath begins with ensuring privacy, informing the client of the intention of bath and maintaining a good conversation. The home health aide should prepare for bath by ensuring the room temperature is warm, door is closed, window and curtains are pulled for confidentiality. Collect all the equipment and materials to include: big pan or bowl, two firm chairs, soap and soap dish, bathing cloth, towels, a plastic covering for protection of chair from becoming wet and preferred cloths. The two chairs can be placed next to the bed, and then one chair is covered with the plastic covering. The soap, dish and big pan are placed on the covered chair. The other chair is for placing the beddings.

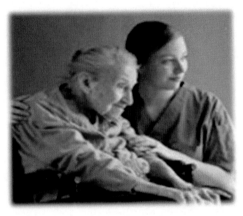

Light covers can be left to make the bed have warmth. The client can be requested to cooperate or assist in removing cloths, from top to bottom. The top can be cleaned, dried out and covered with cloths before moving to the bottom. The body parts that are paralyzed should be the last when removing cloths. The bottom cloths should be slipped slowly from waist to knee to the feet, one side first and then the other side if the person is unable to lift weight. Only the areas being cleaned should not be covered. The water in the bowl should be half full and tested with

elbow for appropriate temperature. The soap should be kept in the dish and wash cloth used as required (Birchenall and Streight, 2003, p. 66).

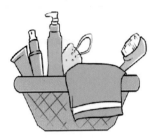

To wash the client's face, the neck and bellow should be covered. Dampen cloth and squeeze out water and hold all the edges before cleaning the face without soap unless requested. Then wash the neck and ears with soap and dry. Wash the arms and hands with wet soapy cloth using long strokes. Then clean the abdomen and chest while paying attention to folds especially under the breast. Wash the front and lower part of body with circular movements and then wash the legs.

The legs can be elevated for access and used with warm wet and soapy cloth using long strokes. Start with hips to knees and then knees to the feet. The feet can be cleaned while paying attention to in between the toes. If the client is unable they can be assisted to clean perennial area. The client can be helped to sit on a towel, by rolling them to one side . The cloth can be given sparing soap, dampened and squeezed. The client can be given the cloth and allowed to clean self. The home health aide should face away as they clean. If they are unable, one should clean using strokes that start from front to back.

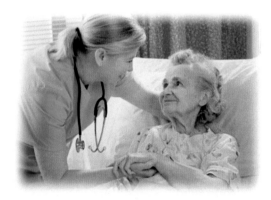

Pay attention to skin folds and dry well. Clean the clients back and remaining sides, from top to bottom and apply skin oil or lotion. At this point one can place the linen on the bed when the client is still on the side. The cloths should be worn beginning with the paralyzed body parts from the top to the bottom. The client should be allowed to choose pajamas or clothing.

Guidelines for lifting and transferring propose that the load should be closest to the body as possible. This allows the center of gravity to be close to the support's base. A wide base for support is considered safe. This means that when lifting a load, one can use the surface close to floor with large base for support.

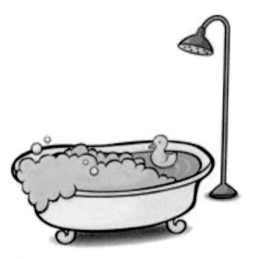

Placing the legs apart creates a wide base for support. The back can be kept straight by bending the knee and hips, while lifting load to lower the center of gravity and use the feet instead of the back. Always move the leg when making a turn and avoid twisting, which can be painful or cause injury.

Proper body mechanics must always be observed when lifting

Small steps are useful in maintaining a stronger base when moving. When lifting load to a position above the head use a stool to step on. Load above the head lowers the centre of gravity (Wernig and Sorrentine, 1989, p. 81).

3. Importance of improvising equipment and adapting care activities in the home.

Depending on the needs of the client Cain (1940, p. 294) suggests that, different equipment may be improvised because of cost and safety in their use. An example is the use of plastic chairs in bathing. The plastic chairs are affordable and easy to maintain clean. The improvised equipment will cut down on cost for extra costs that could have been used to purchase expensive equipment. The comfort of the client is maintained with less costly equipment. The improvised equipment are easy to use and can be applied across all social classes. Improvised equipment are helpful when required equipment are broken or not available. They facilitate the comfort of the client as they receive personalized care. The improvised equipment endorses self-care in the home.

Improvised equipment that can assist in the homecare activities can make a difference in creating good quality of life for the client. The client can gain independence and adapt to changes in their life. Adaptation can make the client feel comfortable and obtain fulfilling personalized care. The patient can sleep well, eat and move in and outside their home when they want.

The availability of improvised equipment and adaptive care activities cause those in need of home health aide come to terms with the progress of their health condition. The activities include rearranging the house for easy mobility and use of when chairs because of weak legs. The client uses the improvised equipment or adaptive activity because it is necessary.

Adaptive care activities necessitate the home health aide to adjust equipment and activities according to the need of the client. Improvised equipment may become convenient and suitable for client when designed for the need of the patient.

4. Personal care delivery at home.

Personal care delivery at home entails giving personalized care according to individual needs of a client. It encourages comfort and safety to the client as they receive care. Personal care delivery entails giving healthcare services using skills while paying attention to safety and comfort of the client. Using the available information, the home health aide uses appropriate skills to deliver care to the client. They skillfully employ communication skills to facilitate their work. They interact with the patient, family and other healthcare professional to give best care as the client obtains healthcare in their home (Shi and Singh 2011, p. 5).

5. Examples of equipment that can be used to provide care.

Equipment used to provide personalized care include: wheel chair for transportation, mobility aids for clients with weak feet, transferring aids, lifting aids, breathing aids, audio and visual aids, incontinence equipment, beds, feeding aids, Hoyer lifts, diapers,

6. Benefits of self-care in promoting wellness.

Self-care is the involvement of an individual in decisions concerning their health. A person practicing self-care is aware of healthcare needs and makes informed decision. Self-care is characterized by healthy eating habits, appropriate lifestyle preferences and being informed on when to ask for medical assistance. Self-care entails making the appropriate decisions to exercise, take a balanced diet, get enough sleep and being kept to prevent any infections that can harm health.

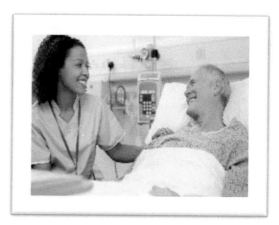

Self-care can cause one to get immunized, treat infections and sickness before it advances, get screening for any

conditions for early detection, follow recommended prescription and getting the correct appointment with a physician. Consequently, a client is able to make correct decisions about concerning their health. For instance, a healthy diet will make the body strong and prevent some illnesses caused by deficiency such as anemia.

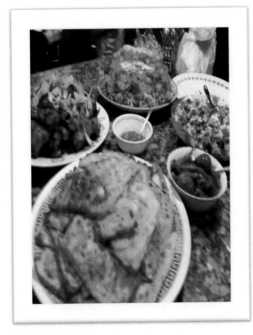

A healthy or balanced diet will keep sickness away. Balanced diet will enable the body to form a strong immune system. Self-care can cause one to choose whether to treat a minor illness at home or at the hospital. It is easy to treat illness when one gives priority to a healthy diet and is able to take their medication as prescribed.

Self-care practices facilitate a good relationship between the client and the healthcare professionals. Communicating with the health care practitioners and the client becomes easier than when the patient is not aware of self-care. Self-care eventually causes one to have good quality of life by preventing and managing illness. Moreover, there is confidence in decision making and hope for improved health (Canadian Pharmacists Association, 2002, p. 5).

7. Key principles of body mechanics.

Body mechanics uses different parts of the body to make safe movement, conserve energy and increase efficiency when conducting different activities with the body. Body mechanics discourage incorrect posture when using the body and reveals physical capabilities.

Body mechanics emphasize balance when performing an action. Unity of action is considered as an important factor in attaining support. All the necessary muscles can be used to give support when a person is moving. The abdomen is considered a powerful source of power. The physical power can also be coordinated with the aid of the abdomen together with the back. The back should be kept upright to give control.

Body mechanics that can be adapted in homecare is to use the correct posture to stand or sit. The chin should be lowed, shoulder rest towards the back and squared. The hips should be above knees when standing up. Twisting should be avoided. When lifting the heavy objects, the muscles in the leg can be used when legs are apart. The knees together with hips should be used for bending while the back is kept straight. The object being should be close to the body.

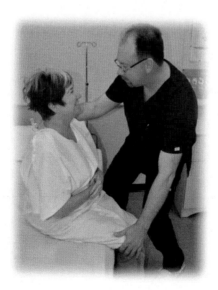

When pulling and pushing, use both hands as well as the legs to acquire force. Use the palm instead of fingers and let the feet be firmly held to the ground when pushing. Pulling and pushing should be preferred to lifting. When reaching out or bending, the feet should be firmly placed on ground and the shoulders apart.

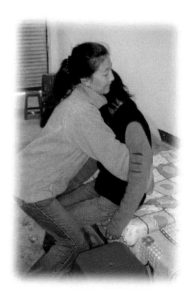

The knees can be bending while the hips should be bending slightly. Avoid balancing or step on a higher ground (or stool). Exercising is another principle that can enable the body performs many functions. The abdomen and leg support lifting, pulling and pushing. When the body is flexible bending is easy. The shoulders give the back a support for posture. Exercising makes the body flexible and strengthens the muscles as Dixon (2000, p. 56) notes.

8. How to adapt body mechanics in the home.

The home health aide can adapt motions that are safe for the client and themselves. This will involve supporting the client when they perform exercise and advice on the safe motions. They may use skills to transfer and lift them. When transferring a client one should ensure that they plan before they act. They should ensure their back is not bending and only lift the person if they are able. They should ask for assistance if the client has a lot of weight. When lowering the client on should spread the legs and avoid twisting.

9. Adaptations that can be made in the home for ambulation and positioning.

The home health aide can ensure that the client gets physical support to sit, stand and move. The client can be supported with pillows when sited. One can hold their hand under the arm and closely to give them support as they stand and walk. Ensure the client changes position after a while to avoid exerting too much pressure on one side.

10. The purpose of passive and active range motion exercise.

Passive range of motions is practiced in clients who cannot do exercise without support. The motions are done with the assistance of a professional to help strengthen muscle and joint with stretching. The purpose of passive range motions is to facilitate gentle movement to muscles and joints for daily movement. The body remains healthy and chances of being completely incapacitated by an illness are lowered. On the other hand, Action range motion exercises are conducted by a health professional to a client who can do exercises without support and therefore only receives instructions for exercising.

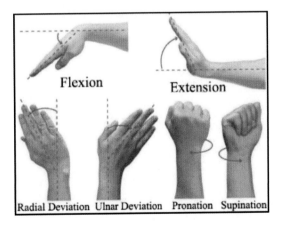

Passive and active range motions secure the muscles from atrophy and enhance circulation. After the motions, the client pain alleviates and they become strong. The client benefits from body flexibility after the exercises.

11. High risk factors for skin breakdown and methods of prevention.

The skin forms the largest organ of the body. A third of the blood circulation occurs in the skin. The skin protects the body from heat, physical acts, chemicals and light. Furthermore, the skin shields the body from infection, maintains good environment and is an important sensory organ. Additionally, the skin retains water, vitamin D and fats that are important. The skin is resilient and can heal after an injury.

Besides being resilient, the skin can undergo a breakdown if the following factors are experienced. When the skin is abused for a long time by friction and moisture can breakdown. A lot of pressure and force will damage the skin. Clients with myelitis, paralysis or illness that cause loss of sensation are susceptible to a skin breakdown. Paralysis affects skin tissue; where the collagen is reduced making the skin

loses elasticity. Additionally, the muscles do not function and the lack of padding could lead to skin breakdown.

Clients who have difficulty shifting weight lack sensation to be able to adjust their position. Their skin can be exposed to extreme heat, cold, discomfort, trauma or sun for long. The client's skin with impaired sensation can be injured from heat near a fire place or a lap top. Ice packs and extreme cold can cause frost bite. Toe nails can in grow and get infected without the client feeling pain. Skin can get sun burns without the client noticing.

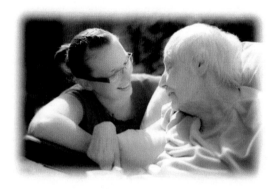

Clients who have impaired sensation and reduced mobility may have pressure ulcers, which is a type of skin breakdown. Other types of skin breakdown reveal as a blister, cut, scrape or burn. Pressure ulcers may affect the bone and sometimes require surgery.

Skin break down still occur even when care is taken and is preventable. Prescribed equipment and care does not guarantee that skin breakdown cannot occur. When the skin breakdown occurs care must be given in the initial stages before it advances. Skin breakdown advances from the initial stages to the advanced stages very quickly (Habif et al 2011, p. 9).

Another factor that can cause skin breakdown is poor nutrition and failure to have liquid food or water. In addition, people who are overweight because of pressure on a particular side if unable to move. Clients with depression or those who abuse substances may be unable to attend to their body. Clients with depression may disregard self-care and neglect their skin.

The skin can be kept clean and dry. Mild soaps can be used for bath, with warm water; since hot water can cause skin dryness. When drying the skin, avoid rubbing and use patting technique. The undergarments should be changed frequently. Pads should be changed immediately after bowel. Adapting to a therapy where the client exercises to strengthen muscles, increase circulation and facilitate flexibility is necessary. Skin breakdown can be prevented by feeding on a balanced diet and taking adequate water. Cutting down on weight will reduce body mass that compress blood vessels. Clients can eat foods rich in Omega three, Zinc, Protein, and Vitamins A and C. The foods nourish the sin and prevent skin breakdown.

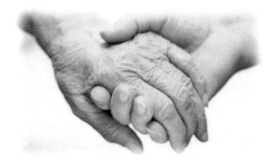

Prolonged pressure on one side can be eliminated by changing positions often. Change positions in bed after around three hours and place pillows at the back. Avoid sleeping on the back if the client had been using a wheel chair. Ensure the client is able to breathe comfortably at all times. Muscle spasms can be managed to allow control by exercising. Straps or braces should be comfortable to avoid pressure if worn correctly.

12. Stages of pressure ulcers/decubitus ulcers and report observation.

Pressure ulcers are characterized by injury of skin or tissue bellow skin from combined friction and pressure. The home health aide should look at the skin to check to check the condition. There are four stages of skin breakdown. In the first stage the skin changes color to red, blue or grey after close to fifteen minutes without pressure, although the skin is still intact. In the next stage the epidermis together with the dermis layers loses skin thickness.

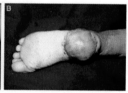

In the following stage, all skin thickness is lost to a depression since the dermis and epidermis layer are absent. In the final and advanced stage the entire skin layers, muscles, bones and tendons are lost. The home health aide can report rashes, turgor, bruises, wrinkles, veins, and bumps. The temperature can be noted whether, cold, warm, cool or hot. Changes that must be reported include: redness or change in skin color, irritation, odor, swelling, drainage, sores and perspiration. It should be reported if the client experiences burning, pain and tingling in the affected skin (Habif 2011, p. 93).

13. Types of ostomies and how to empty and change the pouch.

An ostomy is a surgical opening on a body after a surgery. Types of ostomies include: Colostomy, ileostomy and Urostomy. Ostomies pouch need to be kept clean. The first step to cleaning and changing the pouch is to collect all the materials required to include: another pouch, pouch clip, towel, scissors, wipes, tissue, card and pen, and stoma powder. Changing can be done when bathing. The pouch can be emptied in a toilet. Then the hands are cleaned, and then the pouch is removed.

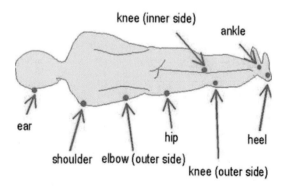

The clip is retained and the used pouch is thrown to a dustbin wrapped in a plastic bag. Clean the area with clean water using a towel and dry it. Inspect the skin to see if it is healthy. Use the wipes to clean around the opening and powder the wipes then gently pat the powder to the skin. The skin should be left to dry for two minutes. Measure the stoma then attach the new pouch using the clip. Finally, clean the hands using soap and water (Hampton and Bryant, 1992, p. 4).

14. Emergencies in the home and critical steps to follow.

Emergencies in the home care include clients who are in danger like fire or drowning in water, and sustained injury from a collapse. It can be faint or absence of breathing from client or unconsciousness. Upon recognizing an emergency, the home health aide should move the client from the danger. If they have fallen and have serious injuries, they should avoid moving them. The ambulance can be called right away. The manager in charge of supervising the home health aide should be notified.

15. The chain of infection in the home care setting.

In the home care setting an agent of infection may be found in the hands, equipment, masks or surfaces. The agent of infection will have a reservoir like a surface, equipment, water, air human where they live. They look for an exit through blood and body secretions.

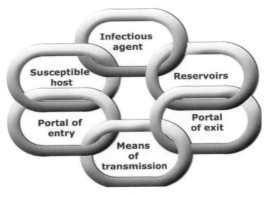

The agent of infection is transmitted to another who has contact with the infected (water, food, air or human). The agent gets entry to the body through the nose, digestive organs, reproductive system, respiratory system, skin and circulatory system.

Chain of Infection

 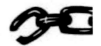

16. Infection control measures to use in the home care setting.

Infections can be controlled in the home setting if hands are cleaned thoroughly very often. The home health aide can take a balanced diet, wash cloths and the body daily. They can get immunized for common infections. Door knobs and other surfaces can be wiped with antiseptic. The mouth can be covered when coughing or sneezing. Waste can be disposed in the trash correctly. The toothbrush can be changed after a few months. Artificial nails can be avoided. It can help for a sick client to stay at home when sick to avoid re-infection and spreading the infection. Moreover, hygiene should be emphasized at all times (Rhinehart and McGoldrick, 2005, 11).

17. Role and responsibilities of the HHA in assisting the client to self-administer medications.

The home health aide role and responsibility in assisting client to self-administer medication includes getting the medicine from the storage and returning after use. Check the labels to confirm the medication is prescribed to the specific client. Observe time and remind the client time for the next dose. Be present as client takes medication and offer help. The client may need juice, spoon and one to open the container. Give support to the hand as the client takes medication, and offer help to return tablets to the container.

18. Conclusion.

Personal care is a significant task in home. Personal care enables the client in home care to be comfortable and prevent infection. Improvised equipment cut down on cost and facilitates homecare delivery. Home care delivery is intended to give the client quality healthcare services. Understanding on body mechanics gives insight on the best way to transfer and move a client. The client needs to exercise for health circulation and muscle strengthening. The skin needs care to prevent it from injuries such as pressure ulcers. The skin

can be protected by eating healthy and
taking care of it. Infections can be
controlled if hygiene is observed.

REFERENCES

Birchenall, J. M. (2012). Mosby's Textbook for the Home Aide. New Jersey: Mosby.

Birchenall, J. M., and Streight, E. (2003) Mosby's Textbook for the Homecare aide, 2nd edition,   New Jersey: Mosby.

Canadian Pharmacists Association (2002) Patient Self Care, Canada: Canadian Pharmacists.

Cain, B. (1940) Improvised Equipment in the Home Care of the Sick, *American Journal of   Public Health and the Nations Health* 30, 3, 294-294.

Dixon, M. W. (2000) Body Mechanics and Self-Care Manual. New Jersey: Prentice Hall.

Habif, T. P., Campbell, J. L., Chapman, M. S., Dinulos, J. G. H., and Zug, K. A. (2011)Skin   Disease: Diagnosis and Treatment, Philadelphia: Saunders.

Hampton, B. and Bryant, R. (1992). Ostomies and Continent Diversions: Nursing Management, Missouri: Mosby.

Rhinehart, E., and McGoldrick, M. (2005) Infection Control In Home Care And Hospice,

        Massachusetts: Jones & Bartlett Learning.Shi, L. and Singh, D. A. (2011) Delivering Health Care in America: A Systems Approach Burlington: Jones & Bartlett Learning.

Wernig, J. K., and Sorrentine, S. A. (1989). Homemaker- Home Health Aide. *Journal of Health Occupation and Education*, 5, 1, 81-82.

CHAPTER FOUR

Nutrition in Home Care

Outline

1. Introduction

2. Key principles of nutrition

3. Potential nutritional problems

4. Therapeutic diets

5. Safe food handling and storage

6. Adaptations for feeding

7. Fluid balancing

8. Community resources for meeting nutritional needs

9. Conclusion

NUTRITION IN HOME CARE.

1. Introduction.

A home care client is depended on good nutrition in their meals if they are to gain energy and strength and restore health. Good nutrition is known to improve the physical body, add to healing and positively contribute to the management of health. This chapter will discuss principles of nutrition, give potential problems for lack of nutrition and talk about therapeutic diet. It will highlight safety in handling food, discuss fluid balance and talk about community resources on nutrition.

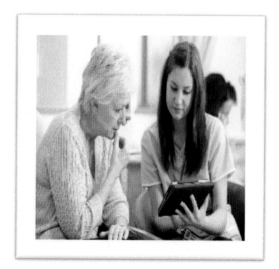

2. Key principles of nutrition.

According to Gibson (2005, p. 25), adhering to principles of nutrition gives the client strength and helps to maintain body weight. It replaces lost minerals and vitamins, boosts the immune and enhances response after treatment. The client should eat a variety of foods from the following groups; carbohydrates, protein, minerals, fats, vitamins and sugars.

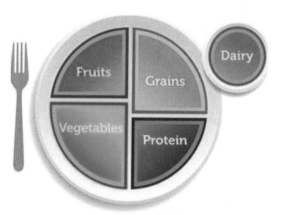

The foods should be taken in correct amount to maintain weight and should avoid dehydration by drinking plenty of fluids. The client can have regular exercise. Three main meals in a day with plenty of snacks in between can be adopted.

Ingram and Lavery (2009, p. 218) points out that, the body is composed of water, minerals, protein, fats, carbohydrates and refuse. Food that is taken builds the body. Food is important in giving the body energy, warmth and retaining heat and energy.

Implementing nutritional principles enable a person to have energy, good health, and reduce sickness. Eat plenty of fruits and vegetables for good health. Increase water intake. Take seasonal foods since they enhance nutrition. Take a wide variety of diverse foods and ensure food is taken in moderation. Whole food nutrition is better than separate nutrition element. Taking supplements is not an equivalent to replacing food. Take food that is good for eating and not poisonous or contaminated. It is important to discipline self to eat food in the right amount. Good nutrition can prevent and at times reverse illnesses. If nutritional principles are followed the cost of care is reduced since ailments subside.

3. Potential nutrition problems.

Birchenall and Streight (2012, p. 19) mention that, home healthcare clients can experience nutritional problems despite paying attention to getting adequate food.

One of the common problems is under nutrition which leads to weight loss.

Weight loss can be easily identified and treated with balanced diet, correct food and beverage quantities. However, medication effects and depression that a client experience can lead to weight loss. The problem is solved by introducing feeding tubes to avoid under nutrition of protein energy.

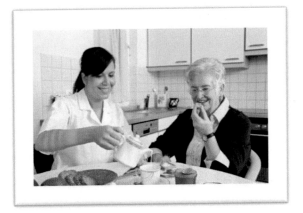

Another problem is deficiency of pyridoxine, folate, vitamin D and minerals like zinc. The deficiency of nutrients hinders healing of wounds and contributes to low immune. Additionally, failure to take adequate fluids causes dehydration. Furthermore, post prandial hypotension can occur and inevitably cause the home care client to have aspiration pneumonia. Aspiration pneumonia can cause a fall.

4. Therapeutic diets.

Therapeutic diets refer to foods that are modified to meet the specific health and physical needs of a client. The modification is recommended by a nutritionist or a medical professional. The objective is to adjust the content of calories, texture or nutrients to the most appropriate depending on the client's condition (William and Schlenker, 2003, p. 17). Therapeutic diets require patience and convincing to the client. This is because they may have body weakness, sickness, lack of appetite or self pity. It is easier to make them understand the use of diet by explanation. Therapeutic diet include food low in cholesterol, food low in residue, regular food, liquid food, soft food, low fat food, food without sodium, food for diabetic and protein diet.

Food low in cholesterol is recommended for clients with heart disease and atherosclerosis. Avoid beef, egg yolk, cheese or food saturated with fats. Food low in residue is best for clients with diarrhea or digestion problems.

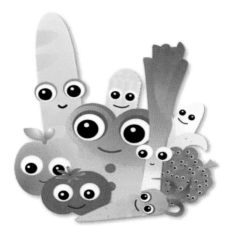

Regular food can be given to clients with ambulatory needs. Their food should have cream sauce, rich desert, fried foods or salad dressing.

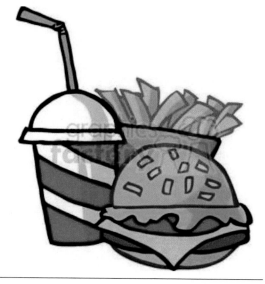

Liquid food is a short term solution for clients recovering from heart attack, surgery and digestion issues. They replace water lost in diarrhea. Soft food is meant for clients who chew little and who have undergone recent surgery. For easy digestion, spicy foods, fried foods, raw fruits and vegetables, coconut, meat or food with tough tissue should be avoided.

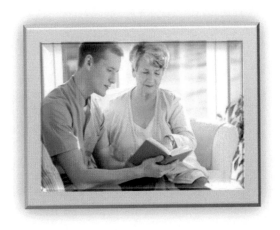

Patients with diabetes mellitus have inadequate insulin and should have certain nutrients according to their specific requirements. They should avoid foods or items rich in sugar. Some patients need food high in calorie, while others need food low in calorie. Client with cardiovascular disease should take a low sodium diet. High protein foods are given to children, pregnant mothers, lactating mothers, adolescents and

clients after burns or infections. Low protein diet is given to clients with allergic kidney disease as William and Schlenker (2003, p. 17) discuss.

5. Safe food handling and storage.

The way food is handled, prepared and stored could cause contamination and lead to sickness.

Food can be a reservoir that can transmit bacteria from one person to another. Food poisoning can be avoided by preparing and storing food in a clean, safe environment using clean water. Safety can be achieved by observing hygiene. Use clean water for cooking, cleaning and drinking.

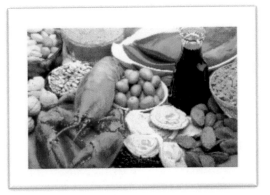

Clean hands before and after eating food. Contaminated water and food is spread by people, pests and pets.

nother safety principle in food handling is separating raw food from cooked food. In addition food should be cooked for the recommended period using the correct temperature to kill germs. Food should be kept away from contamination and at the recommended temperature. Avoid contaminating safe water or cooked food by keeping it covered (William and Schlenker 2003, p. 19).

6. Adaptations for feeding.

Clients need help to feed. The home health aide will be required to feed the client with healthy and appropriate diet. Home health aide should practice patience and avoid rushing the client to take food. Give attention and focus on feeding the client. Feeding time can be used for conversation. They should show interest and think about client. In case the client is able to feed they should be given independence to feed and get support on arms. The client can be allowed to decide on drinks and foods they prefer to feed on.

The client can be allowed to rest as much as possible and get breaks in between meals. Their food may need to be cooked in a manner that does not make them loose appetite or vomit. It is important to be aware of the bladder and bowel movements, to assess if they need more liquids and fiber. Feed the patients according to their nutritional needs and vary the foods widely. Adjust the nutrition as required from time to time and engage the client as much as possible in the decision making when feeding them.

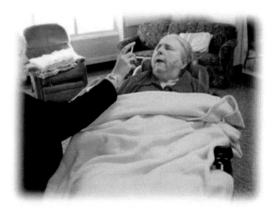

The client may not be able feed orally and this may cause the patient to use enteral feeding. Enteral feeding is commonly known as tube feeding. Tube feeding is given to patients after a surgery or very ill patients. Tube feeding is safe and allows the caregivers to give nutritional supplements. The feeding tubes have different thickness and are inserted differently according to the individual needs of the client. They require monitoring and accuracy in use to ensure the client is comfortable as they benefit from the feeding. Besides using the feeding tubes as an adaptation for giving nutrition, the feeding tubes can be used to give medication (Bradnam and White, 2010, p. 3).

7. Fluid balancing.

Fluid balance entails ensuring the correct amount of fluid is retained in the body. The input and output should be in continuation. Diseases or illness can be a cause of imbalance and this should be considered when handling specific client's needs. Metheny (2010, p. 9) points out that, reduction of body fluid could cause thirst, illness and sometimes death. Fluid in the body changes with the age, body fat and gender. Fluid is lost with exercise, urination, sweating, hemorrhage, vomiting, diarrhea and diuretics. Fluid is retained if client has liver cirrhosis, has high sodium in the body, and has renal failure, if intravenous fluid is given excessively and where there is congestive cardiac.

Fluid balance assists the body in controlling fluid input and output. As a result, fluid balance ensures there is a balance of the hormones.

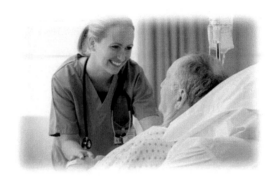

The home health aide may keep the record of weight, blood pressure, respiration, pulse, urine output, tongue saliva, skin thirst, face and temperature in the management of fluid balance. Therefore fluid balance prevents dehydration, and can restore health after fluid loss following an illness. When the fluid balance record is kept, the information can be used to detect deteriorating health. The client becomes comfortable. Thirst or dryness of tongue, sunken eyes and weakness is uncomfortable. Lack of fluid could cause constipation.

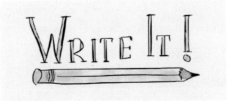

Furthermore, fluid imbalance could lead

to loss of weight. Fluid balance is necessary because the client may be unable to tolerate deprivation from fluid.

8. Community resources for meeting nutritional needs.

There are programs as well as services offered in the community to assist the sick, elderly, children and those in need to get food services. The services aim at meeting the nutritional needs of specific groups like the children and elderly. The Food and Nutrition Service in United States is one of the agencies that help distribute excess food from farms to the needy. The National School Lunch Program and School Breakfast help meet dietary needs of the school going children. Food Stamp Program educates the low income earners on nutrition and gives stamps to the special groups to access food. The Commodity Supplementary Food Program, Nutrition Program for older America, and Head Start Program allows the elderly to get food, education and transport. The programs and services enable the different groups meet their nutritional needs. There are also community programs that offer home delivered meals, social services and home care services from volunteers.

9. Conclusion.

Nutrition in home care contributes to the health of the client. Principles of nutrition require that protein, carbohydrates, minerals, vitamins, sugars and fats be included in a diet. Food should be taken in correct amount and cooked according to recommended time. Adequate water should be taken and regular exercise adapted. Safe and clean food free from contamination or poison should be avoided.

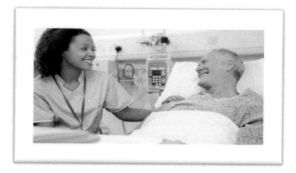

If nutrition is not taken as required the client can lose weight, become dehydrated, get ill, get post prandial hypotension or get aspiration pneumonia. Therapeutic food include: liquid food, regular food, food low in cholesterol, food low in residue, low fat food, food for diabetic, food without sodium, soft food, and protein diet. Food and water should be stored away from contamination. Different clients will need assistance in diet to be able to get nutrition and medication by adapting to diverse texture and method of feeding. Fluids need to be monitored to avoid dehydration or over hydration in the body. The client can get assistance from different services and programs in the community to meet nutritional needs.

BIBLIOGRAPHY

Birchenall, J. and Streight, E. (2012) Mosby's Text book for the Home Care Aide.
Missouri: Mosby.

Bradnam, V. and White, R.(2010) Handbook of Drug Administration Via Enteral
Feeding   Tubes, Illinois: Pharmaceutical Press.

Gibson, R. S. (2005) Principles of nutritional Assessment. USA: Oxford University Press.

Ingram, P. and Lavery, I. (2009) Clinical skills for healthcare Assistants. John Wiley and
Sons.

Metheny, N. M. (2010) Fluid and Electrolyte Balance: Nursing
Considerations, Massachusetts: Jones & Bartlett Learning.

William, R. and Schlenker, E. D. (2003) Essentials of Nutrition and Diet Therapy.
Mosby.

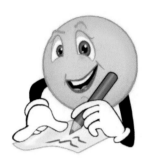

CHAPTER FIVE

Cleaning tasks in home care

Outline

1. Introduction

2. Role of home health aide

3. Principles of safe home environment

4. Procedure, equipment and supplies for house hold tasks

5. Washing and drying dishes

6. Laundering household and personal items

7. Organizing house hold tasks

8. Conclusion

Cleaning tasks in home care

1. Introduction.

Home care entails maintaining cleanliness and safety in the home. A clean home prevents accumulation of dirt which could be a health hazard and reduces chances of getting infection. This essay describes the role of home health aide in maintaining a clean, safe and healthy environment. The essay further talks about principles of safe home environment and procedures for house hold tasks. It explains how to clean utensils, linen and personal items. Guidelines on organizing the household tasks are discussed in this paper.

2. Role of home health aide.

Home health aide gives safety, cleanliness and health assistance by giving personalized care, checking for physical dangers and report to medical authority about the client. By helping in bathing, dressing and toileting they reduce the chances of discomfort and infections (Prieto, 2008, p. 184).

Assistance in movement, taking medication and feeding reduces accidents. Purchasing, preparing, serving and feeding ensure the client remain healthy. In some cases the home health aide educates the client and family which facilitate their cooperation when it comes to maintaining a safe, clean and healthy environment. Home health aide gives support to client and family by ensuring the surrounding is comfortable and can allow safe mobility (Anene 2009, p. 46).

3. Principles of safe home environment.

To maintain a safe home environment avoid objects that could cause stumbling. One can put hand rails or bars in the house for support. Cabinets with dangerous substances and tools should be locked. Allow temperature for water heater to be adjusted to prevent burns. Naked flames should not be left unattended. Moreover, ensure there is an equipped first aid kit and functional fire extinguisher ready and accessible. Communication should be encouraged.

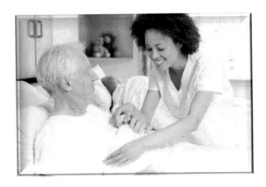

A safe environment will ensure that there is no risk of burns, drowning, chocking, cuts, falls, loud noise, falling objects, broken items, robes and naked electric wires. It may be necessary to implement a system of monitoring movement like a door alarm, bell or supervision. Ensure there is a working telephone in case of an emergency. The home health aide can practice appropriate body mechanics when moving, lifting and transferring client (Birchenall and Streight 2003, p. 4).

In addition cover the mouth when coughing and wear a mask if the client is coughing frequently. Avoid sitting or standing too close to the patient when they cough or have flu. Ensure there is ventilation to allow flow of fresh air. Soiled cloths, linen and items should be kept away from the clean ones. They can be kept together in a room. The soiled

linen can be wrapped so that the soiling is at the middle and does not spill.

4. Procedure, equipment and supplies for house hold tasks.

Leahy et al (2008, p. 17) point out that, it is necessary to collect and get the right equipment and supplies to protect self and to avoid infection when cleaning. House hold equipment and supplies required include: broom, mop, dust pan, disinfectant, bleach, rag, scrub brush, vacuum and scrap. Infection control measures should be considered in every procedure. Wear gloves when performing tasks and handling soiled linen, equipment or cloths. Clean hands regularly, preferably before and after completing tasks. Separate dirty and clean areas. The bathroom should be cleaned with cloth and the toilet wiped with a disposable cloth.

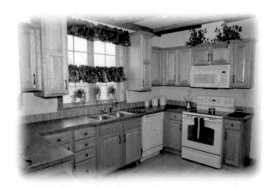

When cleaning the kitchen start with the top to bottom, wipe spills and throw garbage daily. To clean the bathroom cleaning starts from top to bottom then clean sinks, shower and then the toilet. The floor and the water spills should be cleaned last. To clean the living room, begin with vacuuming the carpet. If there is no vacuum cleaner, sweep the carpet with a brush, collect garbage and throw it in a dustbin. Loose rags can then be tacked. Dust and wipe the furniture or items and return them to original place. To clean the floor, sweep first, then mop and finally dry the floor.

5. Washing and drying dishes.

When washing and drying utensils, it is important to establish if there is any utensils that need sterilization. Those that need regular cleaning should be kept together. To begin the cleaning processes gather all the utensils and equipment for sterilization. Get plenty of water, soft cloth and soap. Sort the utensils according to type and dirt. Clean hands and wash less dirty items first. Wash one item at a time. Avoid overcrowding the utensil because it can cause glass to

fall and break. Clean utensils in warm soapy water using a soft dish cloth. Rinse the utensils in clean water, place them in a utensil drying rack and leave them to drip dry for a while. Wipe with a clean dry cloth and place in appropriate place.

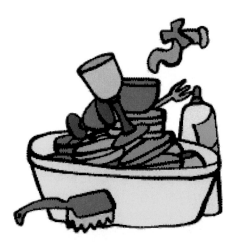

If the utensils were to be sterilized clean and place them in a clean pot with cold water. Place the glass at the bottom and avoid overcrowding. Close the top and heat until there is steam. Let the steam sterilize for the next twenty minutes. When the heat is put out and the steam is no longer there open the lid.

The lid should be open only if the steam has dispersed. Remove utensils using tongs. Keep the sterilized equipment away from the other utensils that are unsterilized (Rice 2006, p. 85).

6. Laundering household and personal items.

Rice (2006, p. 89) indicates that when laundering household and personal items for a client, wear gloves before beginning the tasks. Sort the soiled and unsoiled cloths and linen first. Get information if the cloths or linen are to be washed using a machine and get the instructions on how to operate it. If they are to be hand washed, it may be necessary to consider wearing gloves and using the disinfectant. Empty any contents that may be found in the pockets.

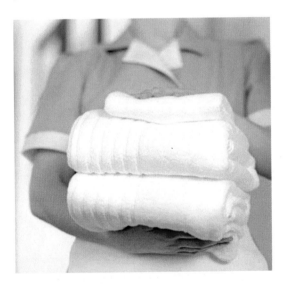

Then sort the cloths and the linen according to color. Some cloths and linen can be cleaned separately if soiled or delicate. Then find out about drying; if to be air dried or to be dried using the drying machine.

7. Organizing house hold tasks.

Household tasks can become overwhelming if proper planning is not done. Begin with a list of household tasks. Then the tasks can be sorted and arranged according to time. Activities can be grouped into daily, weekly and monthly tasks. For example, vacuuming can be done weekly, paying telephone, water and electricity bill monthly, and buying medication upon advice. The rooms can be cleaned once a week. After arranging according to time remove and reduce the unnecessary tasks. For instance, the dishes need more time for cleaning than the fan. Some duties can be designated. If the tasks are too many to handle, one can ask for assistance. This will ensure that all prioritized and necessary tasks are completed. Practice what is in the plan and make adjustments where necessary. When a routine is maintained and adapted household tasks can be accomplished (Gingerch 2008, p. 163).

8. Conclusion.

To create safe, clean and healthy environment, the home health aide practices personalized care and hygiene in giving care. They use body mechanic skills to move patients and educate family together with the client for them to assist in the cooperation of maintaining a clean, safe and healthy environment. Cleanliness is maintained for comfort. Assistance is given in feeding and medication. A safe environment is maintaining by eliminating any danger. The home is cleaned using bleach, a broom, dust pan, scrap, mop, disinfectant, vacuum, and rag and scrub brush. Utensils are washed and dried or disinfected. Lined and personal items are sorted so that the soiled ones are cleaned separately. To organize household tasks, a list of all work is written. The tasks are arranged according to time and the less necessary tasks omitted. Help when there is a lot of work is needed. The plan is followed and adjusted accordingly.

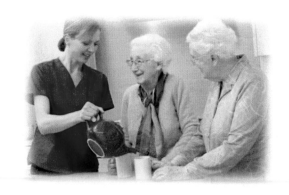

BIBLIOGRAPHY

Anene, E. C. (2009) Home Health Aide Training Manual And Handbook, Bloomington: iUniverse.

Birchenall, J. and Streight, E. (2003) Mosby's Text book for the Home Care Aide. Missouri: Mosby.

Gingerich, B. S. (2008) Pocket Guide for the Home Care Aide, Burlington: Jones & Bartlett   Publishers.

Leahy, W., Fuzy, J., and Grefe, J. (2008) Providing Home Care: A Textbook for Home Health Aides, 3rd Edition. New Mexico: Hartman Publishing, Inc.

Prieto, E. (2008) Home Health Care Provider: A Guide to Essential Skills, New York: Springer   Publishing Company

Rice, R. (2006) Home Care Nursing Practice: Concepts And Application New Jersey: Mosby.

51) All human beings have the same basic physical needs which include:

A) Food and water

B) Activity

C) Sleep and rest

D) All of the above

52) One of the following is not a psychosocial need:

A) Love and affection

B) Shelter

C) Security

D) Self esteem

53) A system of learned behaviors, practiced by a group of people that are considered to be the tradition of that people is called:

A) Actualization

B) Tribe

C) Culture

D) Precision

54) ………..is the name for the condition in which all of the body's systems are their best?

A) Homeostasis

B) Metabolism

C) Peristalsis

D) Arthritis

55) Which of the following is not a system of the body?

A) Endocrine system

B) Diving system

C) Urinary system

D) Nervous system

56) When the outside temperature is too high, the blood vessels:

A) Constrict

B) Becomes excited

C) Dilate

D) Shortens

57) Which of the following gives the body shape and structure?

A) Apocrine and eccrine structures

B) Veins

C) Arteries

D) Bones and ligaments

58) The nervous system controls and coordinates all body functions.

A) True

B) False

59) The taking-in (breathing in) of oxygen by the body is referred to as:

A) Inspiration

B) Expiration

C) Purification

D) Exchange

60) The largest system organ and the system in the body are the:

A) Mouth

B) Skin

C) Esophagus

D) The small intestine

61) One of the following is a common musculoskeletal system disorder?

A) Nephrotic syndrome

B) Histoplasmosis

C) Pneumonia

D) Osteoporosis

62) The digestive system is also called:

A) Respiratory system

B) Gastro-intestinal Tract

C) Metabolic system

D) Nervous system

63) The two major functions of gastrointestinal system are:

A) Digestion and elimination

B) Digestion and locomotion

C) Elimination and respiration

D) None of the above

64) Endocrine glands secrete:

A) Hormones

B) Enzymes

C) Lipase

D) Amylase

65) The sex cells are formed in the male and female sex glands called the:

A) Gonads

B) Androgens

C) Estrogens

D) Lymphatic

66) At age 1-3 toddlers learn to:

A) Choose education

B) Speak

C) Prepare for retirement

D) Develop language skills and vocabularies

67) ……………is a disease or condition that will eventually cause death?

A) A recuperating disease

B) An acute condition

C) Reproductive system

D) A terminal disease

68) The term for the special care a dying person needs is called?

A) Skin care

B) Hospice care

C) Recuperation

D) Advancement stage

69) Which of the following is not included in the normal changes of aging?

    A) Incontinence

    B) Immunity weakens

    C) Appetite decreases

    D) Short-term memory loss occurs

70) Common disorders found in infancy period include:

    A) Prematurity

    B) Low birth weight

    C) Sudden infant death syndrome

    D) All of the above

71) Which of the following are the basic body positions?

    A) Supine

    B) Lateral

    C) Prone

    D) All of the above

72) One of the most important things to consider when transferring a client to a chair or a bed is:

    A) Safety

    B) Nutrition

    C) The Family

    D) Finance

73) Contractures are generally caused by:

    A) Exercise

    B) Driving

    C) Locomotion

    D) Immobility

74) Pulling a client across sheets can cause:

    A) Fluid retention

    B) Shearing

    C) Spinal cord damage

    D) None of the above

75) …………..is a device, such as splint or a brace, which helps support and align a limb and improve its functioning?

    A) Leaning table

    B) An orthotic device

    C) Hand role

    D) Head pillows

76) Hygiene and grooming activities, as well as dressing, eating and toileting are called?

    A) Activities of daily living

    B) Recreational activities

    C) Indoor activities

    D) Unhealthy life styles

77) Oral care should be performed at least:

A) Once a day

B) At bed time

C) Twice a day

D) None of the above

78) ……………is the inhalation of food, fluid or foreign material into the lungs?

A) Expiration

B) Inspiration

C) Aspiration

D) Asphyxia

79) Moving a body part towards the midline of the body is referred to as:

A) Supination

B) Phonation

C) Rotation

D) Adduction

80) One of the following is not done if a client starts to fall during a transfer?

A) Try to reverse or stop a fall

B) Widen your stance

C) Call for help if a family member is around

D) Do not try to reverse or stop a fall

81)……………is the impairment of physical or mental functions:

A) A disability

B) Burn

C) Neuralgia

D) Heart failure

82) A fallacy is:

A) An opinion

B) Truth

C) Being sure

D) A false belief

83) Which of the following can cause mental illness or make it worse?

A) Heredity

B) Stress

C) Environmental factors

D) All of the above

84) Sadness is the only one symptom of:

A) Happiness

B) Depression

C) Hopefulness

D) Excitement

85) Arthritis causes:

A) Dementia

B) Tuberculosis

C) Constipation

D) Stiffness and pain

86) In diabetes mellitus, the pancreas does not produce enough:

A) Estrogen

B) Prolactin

C) Insulin

D) Progesterone

87) Type 2 diabetes can also be referred to as:

    A) Adult-onset diabetes

    B) Electrically-charged insufficiency

    C) Childbearing diabetes

    D) All of the above

88) Paralysis on one side of the body is called:

    A) Hemiplegia

    B) Aphasia

    C) Quadriplegia

    D) Dysphagia

89) Risk factors for cancer include the following, except:

    A) Poor nutrition

    B) Water

    C) Radiation

    D) Tobacco use

90) A brain disorder that affects a person's ability to think and communicate clearly is called:

    A) Anemia

    B) AIDS

    C) Paresis

    D) Schizophrenia

91) Which of the following practices are accepted during housekeeping?

    A) Be organized when performing tasks

    B) Main a safe environment

    C) Familiarize yourself with the household's cleaning materials

    D) All of the above

92) Cleaning of the kitchen should be done:

    A) Once a day

    B) At night only

    C) After every use

    D) Once in a week

93) Which of the following is an example of a detergent?

    A) Soap

    B) Iodine

    C) Kerosene

    D) Anion

94) The process of giving special treatment to items that have heavy soil, spots,, and stains before washing them is called:

    A) Retreating

    B) Escalation

    C) Retouching

D) Pretreating

95) Which of the following would be the reason for changing bed linens?

A) The sheets are wrinkled, making a client uncomfortable

B) The linen was used by another client

C) The linen is damp or unclean

D) All of the above

96) The process by which nutrients are broken down to be used by the body for energy and other needs is referred to as:

A) Reproduction

B) Ham

C) Sausage

D) Orange

B) Metabolism

C) Excitation

D) Lyses

97) There are ………….nutrients needed by the body for growth and development:

A) Three

B) Two

C) Six

D) Four

98) Foods high in sodium include the following, except:

A) Bacon

99) The state of being frightened, excited, confused, in danger or irritated is referred to as:

A) Stress

B) Joy

C) Mood change

D) None of the above

100)…………..occurs when a person does not have enough fluid in his body?

A) Dehydration

B) Fluid overload

C) Crackles in the lungs

D) Water toxicity

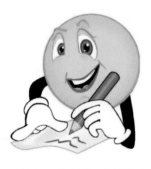

CHAPTER SIX

Prevention of Infection in Home Health Care

Outline

Introduction

Types of infections encountered in home care

Modes of transmission and ways of prevention

Personal Protective Equipment (PPE) in home health care

Conclusion

Although the level and extent to which infection acquired at a hospital during treatment has been exhaustively discussed, measured, and analyzed within a litany of different medical research journals and studies, the level to which infectious disease exists within the home treatment realm is an issue that has received a far reduced level of focus.

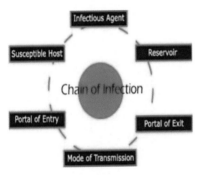

This of course, is because a far smaller percentage of individuals receive home care; however, due to the fact that it represents a growing percentage of the means of health care delivery, the question itself has significance within the context of nursing and medicine. As such, this brief analysis will seek to analyze the definition of infection, types of infection/most common types of infection that exist within home health care, the modes of these different infection transmissions, ways to impede or disrupt such transmissions, and self-protective equipment and its application within the home health care setting.

Though home health care accounts for but a small percentage of total health care delivery within the United States, it is nonetheless a growing sector of health care deserves discussion. According to a recent study, there has been a high level of growth within home care; however, it still pales in comparison to the total amount of money that is expended upon hospital care. As of 2011, home care represented just 3% of total health care expenditures as compared to over 31% of total expenditure taking place with relation to traditional hospitals.

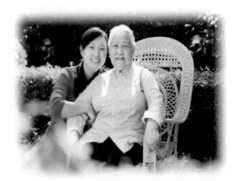

However, the fact remains that even though the figure is small; it is a growing sector and is expected to grow a further 2.5% in the coming decade. As such, it is necessary to understand some of the key nuances that exist within home care as a function of anticipating and treating these issues in a medically expeditious means.

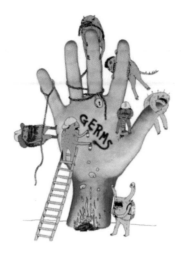

For purposes of this brief analysis, the author will consider infection to be, "the invasion of a host organism's bodily tissues by disease-causing organisms, their multiplication, and the reaction of the host tissues to these organisms and the toxins they produce" (Krismer 2012). With such a broad and encompassing definition, it becomes clear that infection within home care encompasses a broad range of issues; some acting as a more primal threat to health than others.

It is important to note that although many journal entries have warned concerning the level of latent disease and exposure that exists within hospital and primary care, the level to which pathogens exist within the environment of the home is far less uniform. Whereas hospitals most comply with federal standards of cleanliness and procedures for disposal of an array of disease causing agents, regularly schedule cleanings, and a host of other preventative mechanisms, home care is almost invariably not nearly so tightly regulated, or sanitary. For this very reason, the prevalence of disease and the severity with which it affects patients within the given context is almost invariably higher than a similarly community of patients within a traditional medical facility. However, the prevalence of infection within the home care theater is not reason in and of itself to strongly recommend against its implementation as a means of treatment.

Types of infections encountered in home care

With regards to the types of infections and the most common infections that exhibit themselves within home care, there are a number which will herein be discussed. As one might expect, the very same infectious disease agents that exhibit themselves within the hospital care front are also exhibited within home care; albeit, to different extents and total percentage rates than in traditional hospital care.

For instance, studies on home care have typically indicated that the most common types of infections are concentric upon urinary tract infections, followed by an array of different types of skin infections, with staphylococcus aureus, and enterococcus rounding out the least likely but still statistically significant forms of infection exhibited in home care (Patte et al 2009).

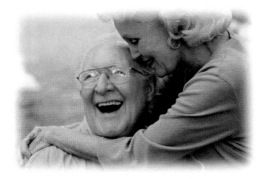

Approximately 6% of the home care patients that have been sampled in different studies have reported infection rates that reflect the aforementioned issues. As a means of understanding the overall prevalence and signs of these diseases, the health care professional can attempt to recognize key symptoms as well as make

the steps necessary to ensure that aggravating factors do not contribute to a worsening of the patient's condition.

Modes of Transmission and ways of prevention

As with any form of infection, the means of transmission can almost always be attributed to contact in one shape or form with a contaminated object or organism. In this sense, the previously discussed information concerning the difficulty in seeking to sterilize the home environment as compared to that of the hospital is brought to mind. Although individuals would often like to think of their home as a superior place with respect to overall cleanliness and presence of disease as compared to that of a hospital, such is not the case. The fact of the matter is that the different disease carrying agents that exist within the home provide for a veritable Petri dish of infectious agents which could negatively impact the health of the patient. Additionally, although the patient or caregivers of the patients may seek to invoke the logic that the "pathogens" that exist within the home are somehow harmless and the patient has been exposed to them their entire life, the inevitable truth is that the patient is in a highly weakened state and likely has never spent time at the home before at a time in which their immune system and overall health are at such a precarious state (Managan et al 2003).

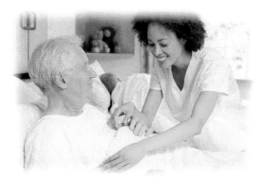

For this reason alone, it is necessary to place a high level of emphasis on seeking to both counteract and prepare for the eventualities that the home care avenue of patient care will necessarily present key challenges that the healthcare professional must differentiate from that of the traditional healthcare model; as exhibited by care within a primary care facility.

Lastly, seeking to ameliorate the risk of transmission for the pathogens that have thus far been discussed within the arena of home care, the practitioner should seek to both employ the same practices that help to ensure that infectious pathogens are kept

at a minimum within the hospitals as well as seeking to impart as much knowledge and best practices as possible to the shareholders within the home. In such a manner, activities that would otherwise spread germs and provide a level of threat to the patient in home care must be sought to be identified as well as reduced or discontinued entirely (Rinehart 2001).

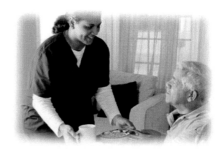

Rather than merely pointing out one or two areas in which the spread of key types of pathogens could be reduced, such an approach requires that the healthcare professional be mindful and highly attuned to the individual nature of the household's that the patient is receiving home care within. In such a way, the healthcare professional will be able to offer insightful advice and guidance with respect to providing as sanitary and pathogen-free a zone of care as is possible.

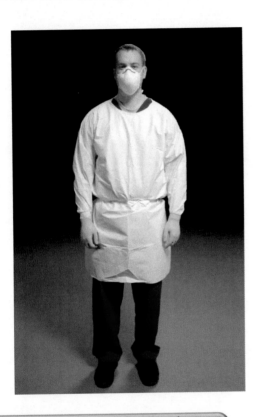

Personal protective equipment in home health care

In the same way, many of the same tools that are utilized within the hospital can also be utilized within the arena of home care. For instance, proper use of gloves, masks, and other pathogen reduction means can be utilized as a means of protecting the patient from pathogens born both within the house and from the outside environment into the home (Weber et al 2009). Although advanced hospital practices such as sterilization of equipment and tools cannot take place within the home, the ability to utilize the aforementioned means as a way to minimize the threat of disease is not insignificant.

Conclusion

Although health care within the home environment exhibits a level of key concerns and dangers that traditional hospital care does not necessarily espouse, the considerations proposed within this chapter help the reader to understand some of the means by which the threats of infection can be lessened through the proper application of key knowledge. As a means of seeking to continually providing a higher level of care, while at the same time providing the end-consumer with the means by which they can take a level of self-determination within the realm of healthcare, it is doubtless that the utilization and application of home care will only continue to grow and expand within the coming years. As such, seeking to understand the key ways in which the medical community can work to sanitize the environment as well as educate the key healthcare shareholders in the process has a direct effect on the overall efficacy of the process.

REFERENCES

Krismer, M. (2012). Definition of infection. *Hip International*, S2-S4.
doi:10.5301/HIP.2012.9563

Manangan, L. P., Pearson, M. L., Tokars, J. I., Miller, E., & Jarvis, W. R. (2003).
National Surveillance of Healthcare-Associated Infections in Home Care Settings
-- Feasible or Not?. *Journal Of Community Health Nursing*, *20*(4), 223-231.

Patte, R., Drouvot, V., Quenon, J., Denic, L., Briand, V., & Patris, S. (2005). Prevalence
of hospital-acquired infections in a home care setting. *Journal Of Hospital
Infection*, *59*(2), 148-151.

Rhinehart, E. (2001). Infection Control in Home Care. *Emerging Infectious Diseases*,
7(2), 208.

Weber, D., Brown, V., Huslage, K., Sickbert-Bennett, E., & Rutala, W. (2009). Device-
related infections in home health care and hospice: infection rates, 1998-2008.
Infection Control & Hospital Epidemiology, *30*(10), 1022-1024.
doi:http://dx.doi.org/10.1086/605641

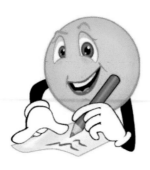

Chapter 7

Vital Signs

Vital signs can reflect the functions of three body processes necessary for life:

Body temperature

Respiration

Heart function

The four vital signs of body function are:

Temperature

Pulse

Respiration

Blood pressure

Vital Signs

Reflect the functions of three body processes necessary for life:

1 Body temperature

2 Respiration

3 Heart function

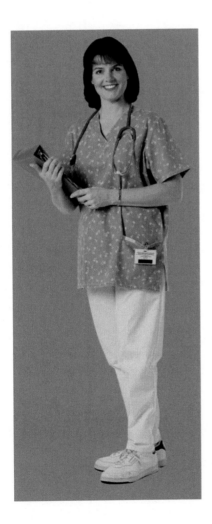

The four vital signs of body function are:

 Temperature

 Pulse

 Respiration

 Blood Pressure

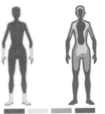

Body temperature is a balance between heat production and heat loss in conjunction with each other, maintained and regulated by the hypothalamus.

Thermometers are used to measure temperature using the Fahrenheit and Centigrade or Celsius scale. Temperature sites are the following: mouth, rectum, ear (tympanic membrane), and the axilla (underarm). The normal ranges for each site are:

+ Site   Normal Range
+ Rectal   98.6Fto 100.6F (37.0C to 38.1C)
+ Oral   97.6F to 99.6F (36.5C to 37.5C)
+ Axillary 96.6F to 98.6F (35.9C to 37.0C)
+ Tympanic Membrane   98.6F 37C)

Some terms used to describe body temperature are:

Febrile – presence of fever

Afebrile – absence of fever

Fever – elevated body temperature beyond normal range. Types of fever are:

Intermittent: fluctuating fever that returns to or below baseline then rises again.

Remittent: fluctuating fever that remains elevated; it does not return to baseline temperature.

Continuous: a fever that remains constant above the baseline; it does not fluctuate.

Oral temperature is the most common method of measurement; however, it is not taken from the following patients:

➢ infants and children less than six years old
➢ patients who has had surgery or facial, neck, nose, or mouth injury
➢ those receiving oxygen
➢ those with nasogastric tubes
➢ patients with convulsive seizure
➢ hemiplegic patients
➢ patients with altered mental status

Wait for 30 minutes to take the oral temperature in patients who have just finished eating, drinking, or smoking. When taking the temperature, leave the thermometer in the patient's mouth for 3-5 minutes or as required by agency policy.

Rectal temperature is taken when oral temperature is not feasible. However, it is not taken from the following patients:
✓ patients with heart disease
✓ patients with rectal disease or disorder or has had rectal surgery
✓ patients with diarrhea

It is taken with the patient in a side-lying position and the thermometer and the patient's hip is held throughout the procedure so the thermometer is not lost in the rectum or broken.

Axillary temperature is the least accurate and is taken only when no other temperature site can be used. The axilla, (the underarm) should be clean and dry and the thermometer should be held in place for 5-10 minutes or as required by the facility policy.

Tympanic temperature is useful for children and confused patients because of the speed of operation of the tympanic thermometer. A covered probe is gently inserted into the ear canal and temperature is measured within seconds (1–3 seconds). It is not used if the patient has an ear disorder or ear drainage.

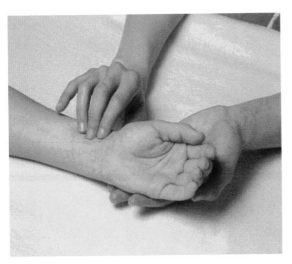

PULSE

The normal adult pulse rate ranges between 60 and 100 beats per minute. The site most commonly used for taking pulse is the radial artery found in the wrist on the same side as the thumb. It is felt with the first two or three fingers (never with the thumb) and usually taken for 30 seconds multiplied by two to get the rate per minute. If the rate is unusually fast or slow, however, count it for 60 seconds.

The apical pulse is a more accurate measurement of the heart rate and it is taken over the apex of the heart by auscultation using the stethoscope. It is used for patients with irregular heart rate and for infants and small children.

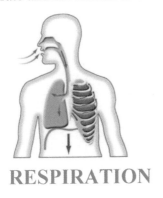

RESPIRATION

When measuring respiration, respiratory characteristics such as rate, rhythm, and depth are taken into account. Rate is the number of respirations per minute. The normal range for adults is 12 to 20 per minute. One inspiration (inhalation) and one expiration (exhalation) counts as one respiration. It is counted for 30 seconds multiplied by two or for a full minute.

Some rate abnormalities are the following:

Apnea – This is a temporary complete absence of breathing which may be a result of a reduction in the stimuli to the respiratory centers of the brain.

Tachypnea – This is a respiration rate of greater than 40/min. It is transient in the newborn and maybe caused by the hysteria in the adult.

Bradypnea – decrease in numbers of respirations. This occurs during sleep. It may also be due to certain diseases.

Respiratory rhythm refers to the pattern of breathing. It can vary with age: infants have an irregular rhythm while adults have regular.

Some abnormalities in the rhythm are the following:

 Cheyne-Stokes – this is a regular pattern of irregular breathing rate.

Orthopnea – this is difficulty or inability to breath unless in an upright position.

Depth of respiration refers to the amount of air that is inspired and expired during each respiration. Some abnormalities in the depth of respirations are the following:

Hypoventilation: state in which reduced amount of air enters the lungs resulting in decreased oxygen level and increased carbon dioxide level in blood. It can be due to breathing that is too shallow, or too slow, or to diminished lung function.

Hyperpnea: abnormal increase in the depth and rate of breathing. *Hyperventilation*: state in which there is an increased amount of air entering the lungs.

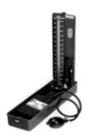

BLOOD PRESSURE

This is the measurement of the amount of force exerted by the blood on the peripheral arterial walls and is expressed in millimeters (mm) of mercury (Hg). The measurement consist of two components: the highest (systole) and lowest (diastole) amount of pressure exerted during the cardiac cycle.

A stethoscope and sphygmomanometer of either aneroid or mercury type are used. The size of the cuff of the sphygmomanometer will depend on the circumference of the limb and not the age of the patient. The width of the inflatable bag within the cuff should be about 40% of this circumference – 12 cm to 14 cm in an average adult. The length of the bag should be about 80% of this circumference – almost long enough to encircle the arm. Cuffs that are too short or narrow may give falsely high readings, e.g. a regular cuff on an obese arm may lead to a false diagnosis of hypertension.

The inflatable bag is centered over the brachial artery with the lower border about 2.5cm above the antecubital crease. The cuff is positioned at heart level. If the brachial artery is far below the heart level the blood pressure will appear falsely high. If the brachial artery is far above heart level, blood pressure will appear falsely low.

Blood pressure is taken by determining first the palpatory systolic pressure over the brachial artery. Then with the bell of the stethoscope over the brachial artery, the cuff is inflated again to about 30 mm Hg above the palpatory systolic pressure and deflated slowly, allowing the pressure to drop at a rate of about 2 to 3 mmHg per second. Note the level at which you hear the sounds of at least two consecutive beats. Blood pressure is taken by determining first the palpatory systolic pressure over the brachial artery.

Then with the bell of the stethoscope over the brachial artery, the cuff is inflated again to about 30 mm Hg above the palpatory systolic pressure and deflated slowly, allowing the pressure to drop at a rate of about 2 to 3 mmHg per second. Note the level at which you hear the sounds of at least two consecutive beats.

This is the systolic pressure. Continue to lower the pressure slowly until the sounds become muffled and then disappear. Then deflate the cuff rapidly to zero. The disappearance point, which is usually only a few mmHg below the muffling point, marks the generally accepted diastolic pressure. Both the systolic and diastolic pressure levels are read the nearest 2 mmHg.

Common errors in blood pressure measurements:

Improper cuff size. Cuffs that are too short or narrow may give falsely high readings. Using a regular cuff on an obese arm may lead to a false diagnosis of hypertension. For an obese arm, select a cuff with a larger than standard bag.

The arm is not at heart level. If the brachial artery is much below the heart level, the blood pressure will appear falsely high. Conversely, if the artery is much above heart level, blood pressure will appear falsely low. A 13.6 cm difference between arterial and cardiac levels produces a blood pressure error of 10mmHg.

Cuff is not completely deflated before use. Deflation of the cuff is faster than 2-3 mmHg per second. Rapid deflation will lead to underestimation of the systolic and overestimation of the diastolic pressure.

The cuff is re-inflated during the procedure.

Without allowing the arm to rest for 1-2 minute between readings. Repetitive inflation of the cuff can result in venous congestion, which could make the sound less audible producing artificially low systolic and high diastolic pressure.

IMPROPER CUFF PLACEMENT.

Defective Equipment. A bag that balloons outside the cuff leads to falsely high readings.

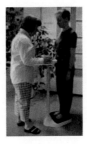

Anthropometric Measurements

The term anthropometric refers to comparative measurements of the body. They are used as indicators of the state of health and well-being of the patient and are often included in the initial measurement of vital signs. Anthropometric measurements require precise measuring techniques to be valid.

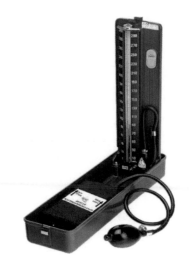

Length, height, weight, weight-for-length, and head circumference (length is used in infants and toddlers, rather than height, because they are unable to stand) are used to assess growth and development in infants, children and adolescents. Individual measurements are usually compared to reference standards on a growth chart.

Height, weight, body mass index (BMI), waist-to-hip ratio, and percentage of body fat are the measurements used for adults. These measures are then compared to reference standards to assess weight status and the risk for various diseases.

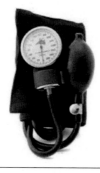

BONUS READING FOR HOME CAREGIVERS

Chapter One: The Ideal Caregiver

"Although the days are busy and the workload is always growing, there are still those special moments when someone says or does something and you know you've made a difference in someone's life. That's why I became a nurse."

~Dianne McKenty

Who is a Caregiver?

Those who have had personal experiences relying on a caregiver will tell you caregivers are angels sent from Heaven.

A caregiver is a professional or relative who has committed to look after another. It might be a child or someone with special needs or one who is ill or recuperating from an accident, surgery, or illness. The caregiver may be ministering to the elderly or anyone from a tiny child to adult. A caregiver may be paid or unpaid for his/her work.

The caregiver's duties may be strictly physical if the client is mobility challenged. They might be homemaking if the client is no longer able to cook and clean and needs a companion. The caregiver's duties may be quite different and varied depending on the needs of the patient. Also, the caregiver's duties may change drastically as the client's ability for self-care increases or diminishes.

The need for a caregiver may be relatively short term for a client in rehabilitation or span several years if the client is aging and/or has dementia.

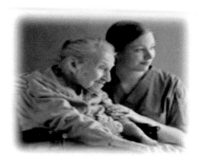

No matter what the age or situation of the client or the relationship or training of the caregiver, all caregivers share common skills, talents, or responsibilities. They include:

1. Knows Responsibilities

The ideal caregiver has a clear idea of what are—and are not—job requirements. These tasks remain the same from one day to another. These tasks might include dressing and/or undressing, toileting, taking the client to appointments, light housekeeping, meal preparation, and other clearly assigned duties.

2. Knows Limitations

The ideal caregiver knows what he or she is not required—or qualified—to do. This might include dispensing medications, giving shots, applying dressings, reporting on healthcare to children, siblings, parents or other caregivers who should not have access to certain information.

3. Carries out the Job Professionally

A responsible caregiver carries out his/her duties reliably, cheerfully, and without funfare. Being a good caregiver is not about getting bouquets or applause. It is about ensuring that the client is well taken care of. Competent caregivers are not in the job for accolades. It's about good care for the client.

4. Maintains Personal Hygiene

Not only does a competent caregiver see to the needs of his/her client. The caregiver also addresses his/her own hygiene. Teeth and hair are clean and maintained. The caregiver dresses professionally and attends to his/her own neat clean and, tidy appearance. Teeth, nails, hands, and hair are clipped and clean. Uniform or clothing is/are clean, well-fitting, and neat.

5. Maintains Punctuality

The competent caregiver knows that howing up on time and being actively present are vital qualities. The client and his family must be able to rely on the caregiver to do his/her job. If the caregiver is not lways punctual, his tardiness results in a lack of confidence.

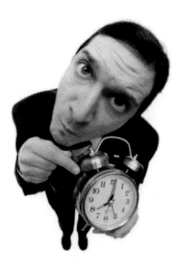

6. Maintains Own Safety

Caregivers who undertake tasks not within their scope of practice endanger the patient's safety and/or that of others as well as his own health. For example: caregivers who attempt to do a task for which they are unqualified (such as giving injections which are not in the job description or lifts which should not be done by one person endanger their own safety as well as the patient's welfare. The wise caregiver does not attempt tasks for which he/she is not qualified or not capable. Good intentions are no excuse for ill-advised actions.

makes adjustments in the client's surroundings to ensure environmental safety.

7. Has Good Observation Skills and Good Initiatives

A competent caregiver possesses astute observation skills. When observing clients' day-to-day health, a reliable caregiver has a keen eye to even slight changes in the patient. He/she takes meticulous, detailed notes and reports these changes to medical supervisors.

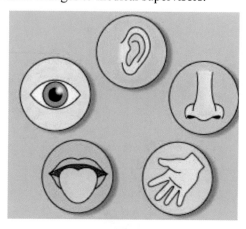

8. IS VERY OPEN TO SUGGESTIONS

Reliable caregivers know the value of supporters. These may be other family members, other caregivers, a caregiver association, or medical professionals. Caregivers who are open to new ideas, new equipment, and new strategies can often find better or less labor-intensive ways of helping clients. Those who are closed to new ideas or defensive when suggestions are made often miss out on helpful strategies or equipment.

When safety issues arise, the responsible caregiver reports these to her supervisor and

9. Has a Sense of Humor

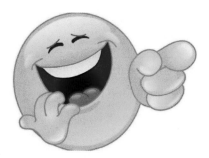

If you choose to enjoy the humorous moments presented in caregiving it can enliven the environment for both you and your client. Humor often lightens potentially embarrassing situations for you and the patient. Even in dire circumstances, it is helpful to laugh. Whether you are a professional or someone who has been pressed into becoming a caregiver for a friend, neighbor, or family member, you will find a sense of humor essential. Having an upbeat attitude can put a positive light on the challenges and trials of caregiving.

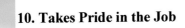

10. Takes Pride in the Job

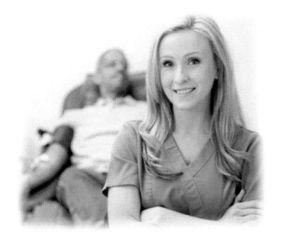

Caregivers who take pride in the service they provide make life easier for themselves and their clients. Caregiving can be tedious. But, caregivers perform a meaningful and vital job. They offer a quality of life to their patients and the family. Without them, life for those people would be vastly different.

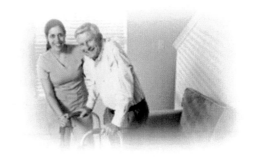

Chapter Two: Care of the Elderly Patient

The closest thing to being cared for is to care for someone else.

~Carson McCullers

Caregiving of elderly patients is on the rise. Many seniors are finding that hiring a caregiver is a cost-effective alternative to living in an extended care facility. Moreover, they do not need the intensive and ongoing care that such a facility affords and they like the option of living in their own home. As the population of seniors continues to increase and as many seniors are living longer, there are increasing employment opportunities for those who wish to work with seniors in individual homes or in institutions.

Because seniors are a unique population, caregivers need to be aware of specific safety concerns. As seniors age, home becomes an increasingly dangerous place for them. Almost two and a half million accidents in USA alone occur to seniors in their homes. Seniors often resist institutional settings, preferring instead to live in their own homes. Most of these homes were not designed for senior living and have not been renovated to accommodate senior limitations. The number one cause of senior accidents in their homes is falls. A third of seniors sustain a fall annually. Over seven thousand US seniors die each year from falls.

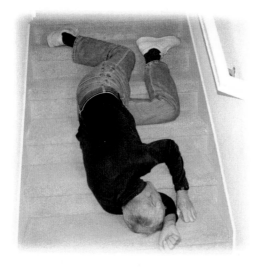

Caregivers need to be vigilant about fall possibilities and take safety precautions to offset diminished senior mobility capacity caused by poorer vision, less acute hearing, mobility and cognitive problems.

- Solutions range from simple to complex: strengthening and balance exercises are a help. "Fall safe" clinics are a good way to guard against sustaining injuries from a fall. Installing grab bars in areas around toilet and tub in the bathroom are good preventative measures. Ambulation training and use of canes and walkers is also good in preventing falls.

- Look at potential fall obstacles like mats and rugs and remove them. Repair frayed carpet, tape or tack down loose rug edges.

- Look at furniture arrangements. Change them to allow safe walking between the furniture within all rooms in the house. If a walker or cane is being used in the house, make sure the path is wide enough to prevent cane or wheels to catch on furniture.

- If your client uses oxygen, make sure no one smokes. Avoid all open flame sources including fireplaces, stoves, candles and oil lamps.

- Unplug appliances when they are not being used. Tuck cords away and secure with elastic bands so they do not hang down or get caught on anything.

- Make sure you and your patient wear close-fitting sleeves. Long and/or loose sleeves can get caught and cause spills, scalds, and burns

- If something spills, clean it up immediately. Sticky, slippery or even wet spots can cause slips and falls.

- Never allow your senior patient to stand on chairs or stools to reach things in higher shelves or cupboards.

- Buy a gripper for those higher and lower objects so your senior client does not have to reach up or down for things, preventing a fall caused by lack of balance.

- The bathroom is the most common location for falls. Make it safe! Place non-skid mat in bathtub/shower. Install grab bars. Consider a walk shower or a step-in bathtub.

- Keep closet doors and drawers closed to prevent falls, bruises, or tripping.

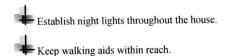
Establish night lights throughout the house.

Keep walking aids within reach.

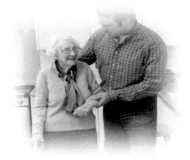

Caregivers who specialize in working with the elderly need an understanding of the physical, psychological and social traits of elderly patients which make them unique. For example: Geriatric clients have aging bodies that are different from younger clients. Various organ systems have declined. Health issues change. Lifestyle choices narrow. Symptoms that would have been brushed off as minor irritations in earlier life become major hurdles and fearsome in their importance to an elderly body.

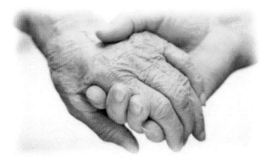

Lifestyle choices seniors made earlier in life come back to haunt them in their senior years: smoking, drinking, overeating, lack of exercise which may not have seemed to affect youthful

bodies now take their toll on aging constitutions in the form of respiratory failure, liver failure, diminished lung capacity, heart disease and mobility issues among others.

Seniors may have social issues. Many of their friends may be gone. They may not have the stamina or mobility to get out to events, hobbies, social circles and other opportunities for being with others. Many seniors suffer loneliness and depression because of a lack of social stimulation. The physical and social problems of a senior patient will naturally be challenges to a caregiver of seniors.

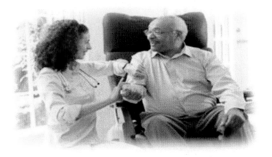

Caregivers who work with the elderly have special challenges and rewards.
The elderly are a unique group. They possess certain character traits which make them frustrating and yet a joy to serve. No matter how you look at it, working with the elderly is a unique experience. What makes them unique?

1. **The Elderly Hates to Seek Assistance**

There is any number of explanations for their reluctance to ask for help. Some of them are convinced they can do it themselves. Others hate to give up yet another part of their independence. Some think it makes them look weak or incompetent. Many don't want others to know how dependent they have become. Some are too embarrassed to ask for assistance.

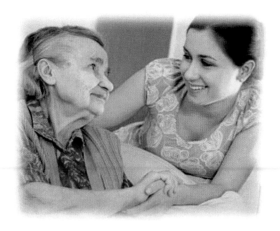

Be ready to step in when you see a potential danger. That is the time to just do it and not ask.

Because all those feelings are rattling around in a senior's head, it is vital that you as a caregiver be diplomatic about doing things. Loosen bottle caps. Cut meat before it is served. Remove those pesky tops from yogurt and pudding cups. Prepare coffee with cream and sugar the way the senior likes it before it reaches the table or tray.

If you know ahead that something will be a challenge, try to avoid those awkward moments by stepping up and offering an arm or moving things before they become obstacles or safety issues.

1. **Elderly May Have Dementia Issues**

Working with the memory challenged is as difficult for the senior as it is for the caregiver. Sometimes the patient may not even know who you are. This gives rise to all sorts of problems including terror, violent reactions, evasion, stubborn refusal to co-operate and fleeing.

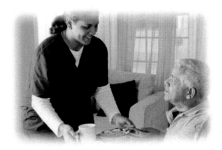

The lack of recognition of the memory challenged means they often do not understand that you are there to help them. Unlimited amounts of patience, empathy, understanding and good humor are required to deal with these situations. Your quiet, pleasant, consistent attitude will reap benefits. If you remain calm and act with resolve, they may eventually remember you and why you are there.

Posting signs and notes and pictures helps the memory challenged make connections. Going over these things with each visit also helps with short-term memory.

2. Seniors Require Higher Levels of Personal Care

One of the unique needs of seniors is that they frequently require more personal care as they age.

Caregivers need training in the best ways to assist seniors in such areas as bathing, dressing, foot care, toileting. Remember: The best strategies for assisting one individual may not work with another. Be prepared with a bag of tricks.

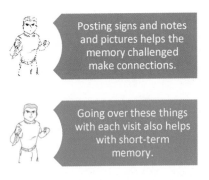

Posting signs and notes and pictures helps the memory challenged make connections.

Going over these things with each visit also helps with short-term memory.

Empathize with those who cannot perform personal care that you take for granted and do effortlessly. Be patient in the face of their frustration, embarrassment and even irritability. Instead of being hurt at their abruptness or demands, be patient and good humored.

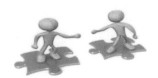

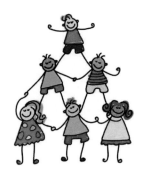

3. There's a Special Bond

Attachment to your patient often occurs when you work with seniors. While this emotional bond can be positive, as a caregiver, you need to keep your professional distance for the well-being of both you and the senior you are caring for. When you develop an emotional link, you are often tempted to do more for your patient than you are required to do or should be doing professionally. If you become too attached there is also the issue of the anguish you will suffer watching them deal with challenges like lack of mobility, dementia, arthritis that are a natural bane of growing old.

When an attachment beyond patient-caregiver develops, you may have trouble with death. Because a bond develops it is crucial that you, as the caregiver, receive counselling in navigating attachment and/or grief issues.

Having a support group of people who are family members caring for seniors and/or professional caregivers whose clients are seniors is often helpful. These people recognize the unique challenges of working with seniors and may be able to offer solutions as well as emotional support.

It may even be that you will, at some point need to consider providing care for a different age group or a career change due to burn out. It takes a special type of person to work with seniors on an ongoing basis.

Typical Duties of Caregivers of the Elderly

If you have an elderly patient, it is not unlikely that you will be called upon to fulfill any or all of the following duties:

a) **Prepare meals or assist with meal preparation**

b) **Shop for groceries, medications**

c) **Complete banking duties, pay bills**

d) **Assist with transfers to and from bed, bath, toilet**

e) **Light housekeeping of client's home: laundry, tidying up, trash collection, dishwashing,**

f) **Keep family informed of patient's progress**

g) **Liaison with other service people who serve this patient**

h) **Prepare medications and offer these to patient**

i) **Transport patient to and from medical appointments, shopping, social events**

j) **Effective communication with client, family, neighbors, community service agencies**

k) **Organize appointments, paperwork, keep track of patient's schedule**

l) **Ensure client is in a safe environment**

m) **Provide social interaction through discussion, activities, social outings for the elderly patient.**

Tips for Caregiving with Elderly Clients

Here are some tips that have helped to deal more effectively with clients and elderly family members.

1. Get Training

There is no replacement for good training. When I look back on how I cared for my first clients, I cringe. I was enthusiastic and pleasant. But I was ill equipped to assist the seniors whom I served. I didn't have the strategies and skills I now possess. My advice is: Get all the training that is offered. Take courses. Attend seminars. Talk with others experienced in the field of senior care. Never miss an opportunity to learn about new equipment, new strategies, new research in the field of caring for the elderly. The National Caregiver Certification Association offers great training courses for caregivers. www.thencca.com

2. Be Ready for the Next Step

Elder care is often fraught with crises as seniors encounter new health challenges. An occupational therapist once told me, "Always plan for two steps ahead because, by the time you've set the next step in place, you are frequently past that one already."

Whether you are a family member or a professional caregiver, you need to be prepared for new situations which will demand new and different types of care. Therefore, knowing the road ahead and what can—and frequently will—happen means you are more prepared to deal with what's ahead. It's rather like plotting a trip route but having alternatives in case of heavy traffic, construction, bad weather, or other contingencies. Your time with an elderly patient will go smoother if you keep a 'weather eye' on that journey. More on observation and record keeping later.

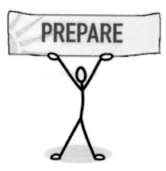

Know how to access support services. Learn what is available through such sources as AgingCare.com and Medicare.gov. Because we are an aging population, many new websites exist. Others have added more helpful information on services for seniors.

3. Set Reasonable Boundaries

For your own physical and emotional safety, you need to set boundaries. Seniors can be demanding. Others resist help. It is important to you physically, emotionally, and legally that you set realistic boundaries. You cannot do lifting single handedly if it is unsafe to you and/or to your client. You cannot be on duty 24/7. If you allow this to occur, you will not be able to offer quality care when you are needed.

Setting healthy physical and emotional boundaries does not make you selfish. You have to balance client needs with your own.

Boundaries remind both you and the senior that yours is a professional relationship. It highlights the expectations of each of you towards the other. Boundaries nurture mutual respect and autonomy in your patient-caregiver relationship. If you are a family member, establishing this boundary is even more critical. From the outset, establish clear boundaries you can both agree upon and be consistent about sticking to them.

4. Encourage Patient Independence

Seniors should be encouraged to do all they can for themselves. There are many ways a caregiver can help seniors maintain their independence as much as possible without endangering their health or being punitive. Here are some things to consider in nurturing the independence of elderly clients.

a) Safety First

Senior independence should always be based on their staying safe. Things to consider in "safeguarding" a home so seniors can move about independently include:

- Removing rugs, furniture, etc. which presents potential mobility challenges
- Making sure there is adequate lighting for clear vision of the path both indoors and out
- Dealing with uneven floor levels

- Ensuring steps have solid handrails on both sides or are ramped. Installation of a stair chair might also be a solution to relocation.

- Removing potential dangers in the kitchen. This might include an automatic shut off or disabling the stove.

- Easy location of fire extinguisher and smoke/CO detectors in good working order. Make sure your patient knows how to use the fire extinguisher and how to contact the fire department.

- Life line or Medical Alert system in case of falls

- Wherever possible, having bathroom, bedroom, kitchen, and living areas on one floor

- Bathrooms are the site of 80% of senior falls. Safeguards include raised toilets with arm rails, removing any mats, installing skip-resistant mats in the tub, installing grab bars for easy access in and out of the tub or shower, removing glass containers, and perhaps a handheld shower head and a bath chair.

- Streamlining seniors' access to mail, newspaper and other deliveries to prevent falls when accessing such things. For example

- Consider bedrails for safe getting in and out of bed.

A vigilant caregiver can make an environment user friendly for a senior by noting things that are challenging and planning for making these more manageable for his/her client. The more a senior can do for himself, the better he will feel about himself and his relationship with his caregiver. Have a conversation with the senior client at the outset about his/her abilities, desires, and goals for independence and what he/she no longer feels capable of doing. Then together formulate a plan for care that meets his/her needs and desires. Whenever possible, include children of the senior in a meeting after you and the patient have devised a plan so that everyone is on the same page and no one feels left out.

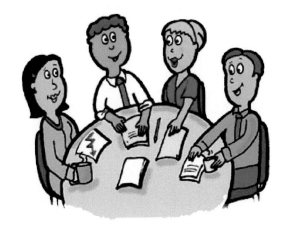

b. Consider Social Links

It is important that your senior client stay in touch with people so he has a happy fulfilling life. These contacts may include: friends, family members, and neighbors. Ways to establish links include seniors' centers, organizations for seniors, hobbies, classes for seniors, and social outings. If your patient is not able to be out, think of ways for these social contacts to come to him/her like a weekly game event, a movie night, Sunday dinner with the family, Skype or FaceTime with friends or relatives at a distance.

Loneliness and isolation are deadly for the elderly. Lack of close contact can raise the risk of premature death by as much as 15%. Ensure your client is not lonely. Seniors who are socially active slow the progression of declining health.

In the computer age, there are lots of ways for seniors to stay connected with family members, websites and chat rooms for seniors and even online games like bridge or scrabble or crossword puzzles.

The fact that a senior no longer drives should not mean he loses the ability to run errands, attend church, go out to dinner, meet friends. Explore availability of association buses, church transit, taxis, and accessibility services for seniors.

Look into what is available through seniors' centers and organizations for the elderly in your area. Seniors' centers often offer such activities are bingo, cards, seniors' lessons and courses, jam sessions, darts, shuffleboard and/or seniors' golf. Travel companies also offer seniors day and overnight excursions. Check out what is available in your client's community through local newspaper, library, and seniors' organizations. It is as important to keep seniors actively involved mentally as physically.

c. Make Technology Useful

As well as performing a valuable link in the senior's social life, technology can be a useful safety resource as well. A portable phone or a cell phone can be a useful tool. You can get cell phones that are easier for seniors to use for calling or texting. This is both a life line and an emergency device. The Jitterbug phone is one model perfect for seniors because it has large buttons and amplified speakers.

Products like Life Alert, Philips Lifeline, and Alert-1 are available. There are increasing numbers of new, easy-to-use safe technology coming on the market all the time. Each enables seniors to call for help by simply pressing a button on a wristband or around the neck device. QuietCare provides monitoring and sends alerts to contact members for under a dollar a day.

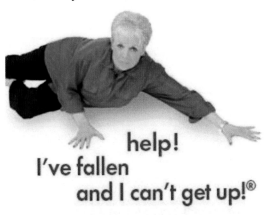

help!
I've fallen
and I can't get up!®

d. Aid in Overcoming Physical Barriers

Don't assume someone confined to bed or to a wheelchair cannot be mentally and/or socially active. There are many activities that don't require physical mobility including board games, crafts, hobbies, genealogy investigations, card games, puzzles, online games, online courses, chat rooms, writing, desktop publishing, movies, TV programs, visits from friends and neighbors, and email.

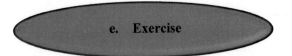

e. Exercise

It's important for seniors to stay as physically active as they can. Look for exercise programs such as Aquacise, yoga for seniors, chair exercises, walking programs, swimming hours for seniors, local gym programs for seniors and stretch classes. Check out what's available in the community. Consider DVD in-home programs especially designed for seniors like "Sweatin' to the Oldies" and "Senior Zumba". Look for programs that are fun and low-impact. Check out yoga programs geared to seniors.

Making regular exercise a part of your client's regular routine helps seniors stay active and make social connections as well. Even small amounts of exercise can help seniors be more independent, reduce blood pressure, avoid heart disease, and reduce the risk of falls.

f. Nurture Active Involvement

It's important that seniors have the ultimate voice in their own care. Nurture decision making in choices of apparel, meals, activities. Encourage phone calls, emails, Skype, whatapp video calls so the patient keeps in contact with the rest of the world. Facilitate visits, activities, and inviting others in on a regular basis. Read newspapers together and/or watch the news and discuss world events. It is all too easy for a senior to get self-centered and tune out what is going on around him. If decisions get made, meals land on his tray and he gets no input, soon he is letting others make the decisions for him and he becomes passive.

These decisions made each day about little things like what to wear, going for a walk, help seniors maintain independence, dignity, and a feeling of control over their lives.

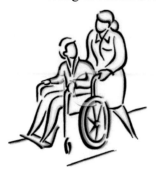

Millions of North Americans serve as caregivers. Some are family members. Others work for homecare agencies. Still others are independent business people. Caregivers who work with seniors need all the skills, talents, and personal traits of caregivers in general. However, they also need some unique qualities which make them an ideal person to work with the elderly age group.

1. Patience

The elderly are often set in their ways. They don't move or think as quickly as they once did and they can also be very self-centred. The caregiver who works with seniors needs to be extraordinarily patient and attuned to these traits in elderly clients.

2. Compassion

When you are working with seniors you need to have an understanding and empathy with challenges that are unique to aging clients.

3. Active Listening

As a caregiver for the elderly, you need to be a good listener, attentive to what your client is saying and inferred messages. Seniors need opportunities to offer opinions and share memories of their life. They need to feel someone is interested and attending to what they are saying.

By being attentive as a caregiver, you will also note physical, mental, and emotional changes in your patient. These changes are often indicators of the need to change services.

4. Dependability

Seniors come to rely on services and personnel who deliver the services they need. It is vital that, as a caregiver, you are there when you say you will be and that you deliver the services the senior needs. Seniors' needs are almost always ongoing and crucial to their good health.

5. Trustworthiness

Caregivers who serve seniors are often placed in a situation where they have access to personal belongings of their clients. It is vital that this trust not be breached and that patients who are vulnerable not be taken advantage of.

6. Creativity

Dedicated caregivers are always looking for better equipment, better strategies and better ways to establish rapport with the seniors they serve. They also look for new ways the elderly can help themselves.

7. Commitment

Good healthcare workers whose clients are elderly demonstrate a commitment to helping their patients retain as much independence as possible while, at the same time, ensuring clients have a safe environment.

8. Good Judgement

Exemplary caregivers of the elderly show good professional judgement regarding patient confidentiality, patient dignity, and patient safety.

9. Attentiveness

Exemplary caregivers of seniors must be attentive to what their clients need and what they should be encouraged to do for themselves. Moreover, caregivers need to be constantly vigilant regarding changes in the client's condition and changing needs of a physical, mental, and/or emotional nature.

10. Good Organization

Exemplary caregivers are well organized. They keep meticulous and detailed notes. Materials, equipment, medications are kept safe and in good order.

Why Choose to Work with the Elderly?

There are a lot of reasons you might choose to work with seniors as clients. There is certainly a ready market for your services. We are an aging population. The need for caregivers for the elderly will continue to increase for the foreseeable future. Those with specialization in this area will be a hot commodity in the labor market. The US Census Bureau estimates that those over sixty-five will double by 2025.

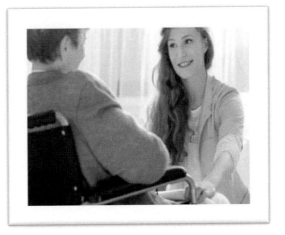

When you work in the field of geriatrics in any area, you have the chance to make significant contributions to other people's lives. Those whom you serve as a senior caregiver are in genuine need of the care you provide. From monitoring health to assisting in personal care, you have the opportunity to nurture good health and independence for the elderly. You also hold the key to making sure your clients have a voice that is heard when their care is discussed.

Caring for seniors is a very rewarding calling. Your presence in the life of an elderly client is most often met with a high level of gratitude and thankfulness by them and their family.

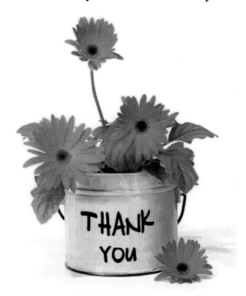

When you work with seniors, you come to understand quickly what is important in life. Many issues or problems that seemed important shrink to insignificance when seen in the light of senior care.
Knowledge of the aging process helps you set your own priorities with greater clarity. It also helps you to dispel your fears of death and dying. End of life becomes an accepted and not unspeakable life stage.

When you work with seniors, you learn a lot. These people have a lifetime of experience and wisdom. They are a treasure trove of facts, strategies and know-how. What they can share when coaxed to do so is invaluable. Seniors have really good stories to tell about what they've done and seen. Working with them can be like living in a soap opera.

➤ Seniors have often cast off their social filter. They tell it like it is and diplomacy not dared. This can be refreshing for those who work with them. Their feelings and reactions are honest.

➤ Working with seniors allows caregivers an opportunity to become specialists in working with a specific healthcare group.

➤ Choosing to work with seniors gives you an opportunity to improve the quality of their lives. This can produce high job satisfaction.

➤ When you care for someone else's mother or father, it gives you hope that excellent care for your parents and you exists.

➤ If you find people in the senior age group interesting and you have respect for elders, you will find a career as a senior caregiver rewarding.

Caregiver Cautions about Working with the Elderly

While working with the elderly as a caregiver comes with rewards, there are some down sides prospective caregivers should consider before choosing this niche market.

Death is inevitable. It's easy to develop a closed bond and hard to watch someone die.

Dementia is a real possibility. In such cases, caregivers can be hit, bitten, spit on, and verbally abused.

As people age, their ability to transfer often fails. Those who are not physically strong often find assisting seniors taxing.

Resistance to Help

One of the problems with working with seniors is often their resistance to medical and/or physical aid. There are several things caregivers cannot do when their clients are resistant.

Why Seniors Resist Help

The first step in working with seniors who are unco-operative is understanding why. Seniors may be experiencing lack of cognitive skills or mental lapses or memory loss. They do not understand or may not trust that what they are being asked to do is for their safety. Seniors may also be angry about the loss of their independence and express this anger in resistance. They may feel that help—particularly when it comes to personal hygiene—comes with a lack of privacy. Or, they may be in denial about their need for medication or physical intervention.

Seniors do not like changes. Offering caregiver support often changes routines and ways of doing things. This adjustment is unsettling and often is met with resistance.

As seniors age, they often become stubborn or outspoken. This manifests itself in resistance to assistance.

Approaching Resistance to Caregiving

In some cases, seeking the help of the family or the family doctor is the best way to deal with patient resistance. In such cases, both family and medical professionals are then aware of the situation and you as caregiver are covered legally.

Before you approach family members or the doctor, you need to determine what type of assistance to keep your client safe, comfortable, and cared for. Making notes and being prepared to discuss what you feel—professionally—needs to occur and where you are meeting resistance. Be specific and descriptive.

Make diplomatic attempts to cajole, nudge, negotiate to get the co-operation of your patient. Record results to discuss—if needed—with family and the doctor.

Listen to what your client is saying. Read between the lines. Ask probing questions. Try to get to the root of the resistance. Ask about patient preferences and try whenever possible to accommodate requests—bearing in mind your patient's safety and well-being.

Take the time to explain why something is being done and how it will occur. Sometimes resistance comes from fear of what they do not understand.

Don't give up and don't take no for an answer. Resistance is intended as a win. Giving up gives the patient encouragement to try again. Be gentle, diplomatic, but firm.

Pick your battles. Sometimes it is better to come at a standoff at another times or using another strategy.

Explain why a procedure is necessary. Ask for your client's co-operation in carrying out your job. Tell your patient the consequences for both the patient and you if this procedure is not followed.

Resistance to assistance is not a news concept. No is it likely to go away any time soon. However, by keeping your patient involved, informed, and seeking co-operation, you may be able to carry out your duties and help your client feel more comfortable about accepting your care.

Chapter Three: Maintaining your Safety as a Caregiver

Physical strength is measured by what we can carry; spiritual by what we can bear.

Studies have shown that the physical and emotional stress of caring for others is widespread. Whether you are a family member or a professional caregiver, you will feel the burden through such things as:

➤ **Increased levels of anxiety and stress**

An aging population that is living longer has resulted in the fact that over forty-four million American adults provide paid and unpaid care for an ever-increasing senior group. Medical advances have resulted in increased longevity. Another result of these improvements is shortened hospital stays and expansion of homecare. Increased costs and care responsibilities now fall on professional and untrained caregivers. It should come as no surprise that these outcomes have resulted in higher levels of stress and anxiety on those who care for seniors in facilities and in their home settings.

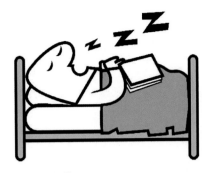

Over a quarter of caregivers admit their job is hard on them emotionally. They feel frustrated and anxious about the lack of progress of their client.

Increased stress has other negative effects on caregiver health. There is an increase in substance abuse including alcohol, drugs, and prescription drugs.

Caregivers with high levels of chronic stress have a higher risk of cognitive impairment, inattention, and short-term memory lapses.

➤ **Interrupted sleep and difficulty getting to sleep**

Because seniors may need assistance during the night and may roam about at night, caregivers often put in seventeen-hour work days. Exhausted, overtired, and anxious about their client, caregivers often have difficulty getting to sleep. Interrupted sleep means that they, like mothers of young children, are sleep deprived.

Almost a quarter of caregivers report feeling so exhausted that they feel incapable of completing their duties responsibly.

Exhausted caregivers have less patience with seniors who can be trying at the best of times. There is a higher risk of irritability, verbal and physical abuse of patients when caregivers are over tired.

➤ **Increased worries about declining health**

Caregivers worry about the health of the client. They are also concerned about their own health. Physical demands of the job, lack of sleep, and worry make the situation overwhelming. They worry about how this stressful job is affecting their own health and who will tend to the senior if they become ill.

➤ **Depression**

Caregivers of the elderly often see their charges in declining physical and/or mental health. Their patients are often depressed or antagonistic and/or hard to handle. Caregivers often work in isolation with only their patient as companion. Therefore, the task—particularly for an unpaid family member—can feel depressing. Studies have shown that between half and three-quarters of caregivers show signs of being clinically depressed. A quarter of them can be classified as having major depression.

➤ **Physical strains of the job**

Working with seniors who often have diminished mobility can be a very taxing job physically. Many clients are no longer able to get out of bed, dress, shower, toilet, or walk unassisted. Caregivers may be lifting patients without assistance from the client or another caregiver.

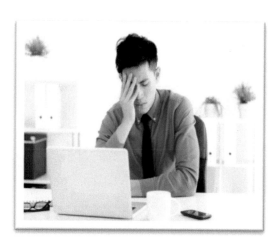

➤ **Loss of Self-Identity**

Caregivers often feel a loss of their own identity, lack of confidence and lack of self-esteem in their role. Because the needs of their client change, they have no clear understanding of their role. They have feelings of being ineffective or unsure of what they are doing.

➤ **Increased likelihood of infections**

Because caregivers work in close contact with bodily fluids and seniors who are often unwell, they have a greater than average chance to pick up germs, bacteria, infections, and communicable diseases. High stress and fatigue lower immune systems. Caregivers frequently forget to wear or do not have time to put on personal protective equipment (PPE).

The Importance of Self Care

For your own health and that of your client, it is important that you look after yourself. Here are some ways to do that:

Give up trying to do everything yourself. Seek resources from associations like Alzheimer's Association. Look into daily and week-end respite facilities in your community, family members, church groups, neighbors.

Visit your doctor regularly. Listen to your body and respond to physical symptoms, stress, exhaustion, insomnia, depression. There is no shame in knowing your limitations and admitting them.

Take precautions against flu and other ailments wherever possible using such resources as flu shots, and current immunizations. Vaccination protects your health and that of the person you're caring for.

Be active. Exercise is vital to staying healthy and as a means of relieving stress and boosting those "feel good" endorphins. Get at least thirty minutes of vigorous movement every day. Choose things you like to do. Start small and build as you become fit.

Make sure to add strength and flexibility exercise to your regimen. You career as a caregiver has a lot of physical challenges. You need to be in good shape.

Fit your program in wherever it works. If your patient naps, it's a great opportunity for you to get some exercise without leaving the home. Consider a stationary bike, yoga, stretches, an exercise DVD.

Involve your patient in gentle exercise wherever it is feasible. A walk in the fresh air or a stroll in the mall is a good workout.

Practice healthy eating for both you and your client. Try Mediterranean dishes with little meat but healthy servings of whole grains, fruit, vegetables, nuts, fish and healthy fats like olive oil.

There are many strategies for helping you cope as a caregiver. Stress can be debilitating. It may manifest as physical symptoms including: digestion problems, hypertension, blurred vision, irritability, eating disorders, lack of concentration, poor judgement. Seek medical assistance. Try relaxation techniques like yoga and guided visualization.

Don't expect unrealistic performance in your role and don't let others place these expectations on you. Focus on the positives. Don't highlight your failures. You will never be able to do everything. Do your best and acknowledge it is your best.

You need a break from caregiving. Make sure you are availing yourself of daily, weekly breaks. You need time for self-care. Use community resources and care options.

It's a fact: Caregivers have a higher likelihood of several work-related problems that other jobs may not have. Let's have a look at some of these.

Because of exposure to patient care, you as a caregiver have a higher risk of illness and infection encountered in such tasks as changing diapers, cleaning up spills, dealing with soiled linens, changing dressings… Your job also exposes you to chemicals found in cleaning products—both in the air and in the environment.

In dealing with your client you may often find yourself in awkward movements and encountering stress from repetitive tasks. Your job also requires lifting and sometimes carrying heavy loads.

Take your breaks regularly	Sleep at least 7 hours a day
Exercise physically	Maintain a sense of humor
	Eat well balanced meals

Because of your work environment and the demands of your clientele, you might be in higher risk of injuries from slips, falls, and trips. You are also more apt to sustain burns, scalds, and injuries from handling sharp objects.

Your job hours often necessitate shift work and/or long work hours which generate issues like fatigue, stress, and insomnia.

Even though there are advantages in working alone, when it comes to caregiving, there are lots of disadvantages in terms of safety and mental outlook.

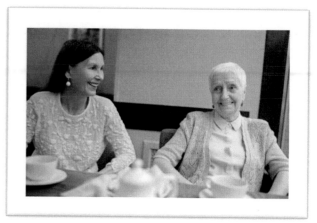

A serious concern for caregivers is workplace violence. Some clients are physically violent. Caregivers often work alone so physical assaults are a reality. Most people think of workplace violence as things like kicking, biting, shoving, spitting, hitting, throwing things. Besides physical assault, workplace violence might include other forms of abuse, threats, intimidation or assaulted in his or her employment. Workplace violence includes:

- Verbal threats and gestures in person, on the phone…
- Property destruction
- Thrown objects
- Written threats
- Harassment
- Demeaning, embarrassing, humiliating acts

- Annoying, alarming, unwelcome gestures or acts
- Bullying, intimidation, inappropriate activities like touching
- Swearing, insults, profanity
- Arguments, sneaky tricks, hiding, sabotage, mind games

Healthcare employees are among the highest-risk groups for workplace violence. They work odd hours. They work alone. The areas in which they work are often dimly lit. Their clients often have mental issues. The job may involve working in high-risk neighborhoods. Emergency response is often slow and not clearly established.

So what are the solutions? Violence in the workplace is not unusual—especially among healthcare professional who are sixteen times more likely to encounter it than any other service profession. The law mandates that workers in high-risk situations be trained in recognizing high-risk situations and intervention strategies. Such trainings include management of assaultive behavior, Crisis Prevention & Intervention, Therapeutic Crisis Intervention, etc. and are available through American Crisis Prevention & Management Association (ACPMA). Their website is

www.acpmaonline.com

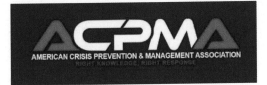

Being alert to potential problems is a first step. Caregivers are advised to conduct an analysis of the environment noting potential areas of health and safety concern. When that has been completed, selecting feasible preventative controls is a good next step. Having a procedure in place for alerting in case of a dangerous situation is also a good measure. The best way to eliminate a hazard is to substitute a safer workplace practice for a potentially dangerous one. This may mean using different strategies for patient transfer or procedure.

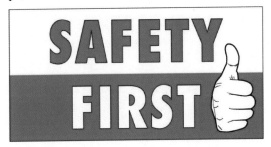

Implementing this may not always be possible. However, often with some thought and ingenuity, you can engineer controls to prevent or control workplace hazards. Such controls may include: setting up physical barriers such as guards, enclosures, or locks to reduce your exposure to the danger; panic buttons; better or added lighting; more and/or accessible exits; closed circuit videography; bulletproof glass. Measures are always unique to the setting and the hazards you face.

Prevention is always the best way to manage workplace safety. If something feels unsafe, you should alert your superior to this concern and document it.

All caregivers need to be trained in protective measures to combat workplace violence.

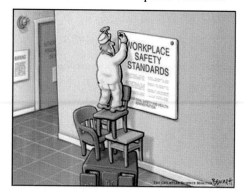

These programs sensitize caregivers to potential hazards and how to protect themselves. Such training also teaches caregivers how to react to workplace violence in a way that keeps them safe and also de-escalates the situation for the well-being of the client. Employers need to ensure this in-service is available and workers take advantage of it. In order to prevent further episodes of worker violence it is necessary for the caregiver to discover why the client reacted and how to prevent repeated behavior.

Appropriate training can increase caregiver readiness to deal with potential situations. It can provide caregivers with the means to identify potential workplace safety areas and thus prevent unsafe practices. It also teaches the caregiver how to address these problems before they arise. Such action greatly reduces the risk of caregivers being assaulted.

Instruction should address any and all potential safety issues in the workplace. Potential threats, types of injuries, problem situations of the facility and how to deal with these should be addressed. Workplace violence can often be avoided or mitigated through information and preparation.

Because caregivers often lift patients who are unable to support themselves, shoulder, neck, and back injuries are common. The human spine provides lift and movement for the human body. However, when lifting or transferring a client, you as caregiver need to give consideration to proper lifting techniques. These will prevent that injury and repetitive movement injuries that occur because of cumulative motion lifting heavy objects.

Lifting is further complicated by the need for awkward physical set ups, working alone, and clients who can be uncooperative, obese, and/or traumatized.

Learning proper lifting technique is vital to caregiver health and safety.
If a patient is being transferred, you should remember to plant feet in a stable position as close to your client as you can. Face your patient. Bend knees slightly. Squat. Hold abdominals in and keep back straight. Make legs take the weight of the lift. By moving as close to your client as possible, you reduce the

back strain. Always try to avoid forward bending. Placing one foot between the client's feet helps establish stability. Lift using a smooth motion rather than a jerk.

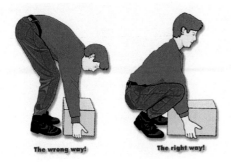

While assisting with dressing, bathing, and lifting, avoid stooping, twisting, or bending so that the spine, joints, and muscles do not get strained. Good training and good adhering to safe practices can go a long way toward prevention on workplace injuries.

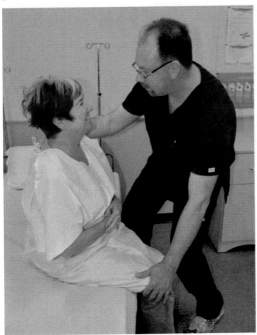

Caregivers need to take health precautions as well as physical and emotional ones to safeguard their health. They may be dealing with infectious diseases, toxic materials and germs as a regular part of their daily activities.

Use of gloves, masks, aprons or gowns should be meticulously obeyed whenever even suspicious materials and situations arise. For more on this, please read the chapter on *Appearance and Hygiene*.

Chapter Four: The Role of the Companion Home Maker

The way to anybody's heart is through a thoughtfully-prepared, beautifully-executed, lovingly-presented meal.

~Leo Buscaglia

A homemaker/companion caregiver ensures that the environment is safe for her client. She keeps the house/apartment/living space clear and neat.

Her duties involve such housekeeping tasks as cleaning, dusting, laundry, dusting, mopping, vacuuming, and other tasks which her client requires to live in his physical setting. She may also do grocery shopping, meal planning, cooking.

The homemaker/companion also visits with the client. She may take the client for walks, attend social, family, and/or recreational activities with the client.

What the Homemaker/Companion Does NOT Do

The homemaker/companion caregiver usually has a high school certificate or equivalent. She can write, read, and speak in English. She owns a car, carries insurance, and has a current driver's license.

The homemaker/companion is not a personal care worker. She does not assist with dressing, personal hygiene, nor transfers. She is not a medical professional so she does not take vitals, contact the doctor, or make observations to healthcare professionals.

Who Would Use a Homemaker/Companion caregiver?

Homemaker/companions are non-medical professionals. Their aim is to help clients remain in their own homes as comfortable and healthy as possible. People who have had surgery or a fall or an illness who would find laundry, cooking, cleaning, running errands presently difficult often qualify for the services of a homemaker/companion. Typical clients may include postpartum mothers and/or those with sports injuries.

The difference between a home health aide and a caregiver is that home health aides are medical professionals, while caregivers/homemakers/companions are not

The services of a homemaker/companion might be stipulated as part of the transition period after a patient leaves the hospital and until he can again live independently.

Most clients are short term. The idea is to help them until they can "get back on their feet".

EXPECTED TASKS

Tasks that clients may expect a homemaker/companion to perform will vary from client to client. They will also change as the patient becomes more independent. In general, homemaker/companion tasks fall into the following categories.

1. Companionship

The primary focus of the homemaker/companion is to provide social interaction with the client. In doing so, the homemaker/companion provides self-esteem and independence.

Interaction may involve talking, board game or card games, reading, taking a walk, visiting with friends and neighbors.

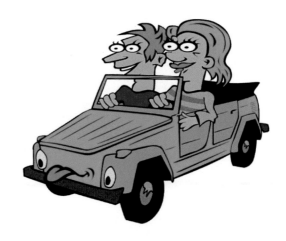

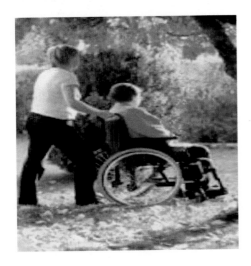

2. Homemaking Duties

This might involve anything required to maintain a home including: dusting, washing, scrubbing, vacuuming carpets and furniture, changing bedding, cleaning the bathroom; laundry, drying, ironing and folding laundry; defrosting refrigerators/freezers; cleaning ovens/stoves and china cabinets; caring for house plants and pets; taking out garbage and general tidying.

3. Kitchen Duties

Grocery shopping, menu preparation, and meal preparation, serving, feeding (if required), washing and drying dishes, tidying the kitchen.

4. Transportation and Escort

The homemaker/companion may transport a client to an appointment or errand with written authorization. She may also escort the client to appointments or errands.

Skills/Abilities of the Ideal Homemaker/Companion

Each homemaker/companion will have different skills/interests/talents. However, the ideal caregiver will have:

1. Active listening skills
2. Ability to work independently
3. Genuine interest in people
4. Enjoys household duties
5. Pride in work
6. Maintains a professional distance from clients Ability to work independently.
7. Excellent communication and listening skills in spoken and written English
8. A compassionate, caring nature

9. Patience
10. Ability to work in a stressful environment
11. Physical and mental fitness to handle the demands of homemaker/companion care giving.
12. Ability to maintain a safe environment for both caregiver and client
13. Good domestic skills
14. Flexible thinker
15. Knows the boundaries of the job description
16. Maintains a safe working environment for herself and for her client
17. Able to react with sound judgement to emergencies
18. Good time management skills

Chapter Five: Positive Communication Techniques

Happiness is an attitude. We either make ourselves miserable, or happy and strong. The amount of work is the same.

~Francesca Reigler

Part of the job of caregiver is effective communication. The caregiver will be called upon to communicate with her client. In addition, she may be required to report to an immediate superior, medical professionals and/or family members of the client. Sometimes, the communication you have with your patient is vital to making adjustments in his care. We'll talk about observation skills later.

Caregiving requires communication with the patient, with the family, and with the rest of the medical team. It's not always easy. Many times your patient may be overwhelmed by his condition and/or medical terminology and/or the sheer number of people with whom he is expected to interact. As his primary caregiver you may have to be his voice.Caregiving often involves providing emotional, social, as well as physical support for your client.

Often, clients feel angry, sad, afraid or lonely. They may not be able to express these feelings.

While they may be incapable of articulating or unwilling to share, many of your patients have fears and concerns about:

- **Changes to their physical or mental abilities**

- **Worries about the loss of the skills they once had**

- **Obsessions about their future**

- **Concerns about becoming a burden**

- **Loneliness because their contemporaries are gone**

It is an asset to the job if you are genuinely interested in people and can show them that you want to hear what they have to say.

Useful communication skills include:

- *Active listening skills*
- *Genuine interest in others*
- *Ability to ask intuitive*
- *Skill at keeping a conversation going by asking appropriate follow-up questions*
- *Listening more than talking*
- *Awareness of body language and facial expression clues to speaker's feelings*
- *Restating what was heard to show understanding of what was said*
- *Noting how other members of the group respond to what the speaker said*

- *Checking for cultural difference in meaning*

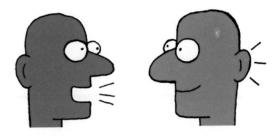

Effective communication rarely occurs overnight. Like most skills it is learned with practice. The following are short practice activities:

1. Initiate short conversations. "What did you do on the weekend?" or a comment about the weather, a TV program, or a sports team is a good starter.

2. Sharing stories about your children or a community project or a hobby with someone who shares your interest is a good way to practice communication skills.

3. Remember: Communication is a two-way street. Think of ways to draw someone into a conversation. Then practice your active listening skills.

4. Provide feedback about your child's experience or a relative's experience with a community organization is a good stimulator

5. Try seeing things from the other person's point of view. Ask questions to help you get a clear picture.

6. Try a variety of communication styles: face-to-face; one-on-one; small group; Skype or FaceTime; texting, email; telephone; memos...Then reflect on which style is most effective? Which most appeals to you? Why?

7. Think about 5 different situations in which you need to communicate. Which style is best in each case? Why?

Effective Communicating Steps:

Communication will be improved if you remind yourself to take these steps in conversation:

- Pause and listen to what the speaker is saying. Then think about what was said. Next, react or respond.

- Follow up with a comment or question to demonstrate your understanding.

- Pauses to reflect what you are going to say or how you are going to react are good! Space doesn't always have to be filled. It is also acceptable not to have a response. You might ask for more information or time to think.

HOW CAN YOU USE COMMUNICATION SKILLS TO HELP YOUR CLIENT?

1. Encourage your client to tell you about his feelings. Use follow-up questions to get him to elaborate. Share your thoughts to stimulate conversation. This will take time. Don't give up the first time you talk.

2. Watch for nonverbal communication. Note body language, eye contact, for clues about feelings and unexpressed concerns.

3. Share your fears and emotions. Let your client know he's not alone in his feelings.

4. Avoid phrases that shut the conversation down. These might be platitudes like, "This will get better." Or judgements like, "Stop complaining. There are people lots worse off than you." Or dismissive phrases like, *"Don't worry about that."*, *"You'll be just fine."* Instead, you need to let your client know that his concerns are understood and acknowledged.

5. Practice listening more and talking less. Give your patient the air time to talk without interrupting.

6. Practice repeating back what your client has said. This shows you understand. Ask for

clarification of anything you aren't sure about.

7. Offer assurance that you will attempt to address your client' physical, emotional, and/or spiritual needs. Demonstrate caring and that you know how to help resolve their issues. Share your plan.

8. Focus discussion on what your client is still able to do. Discuss ways around challenging tasks. Be positive, and encouraging.

9. Always establish eye contact. If your client is in a chair or a bed, sit or squat so you are on the same level. Smile and show active interest in what your client has to say.

10. If a more in-depth conversation is needed don't have it when you are rushed for time. Instead, set aside a time to discuss important issues.

11. Use physical touch in communicating: a touch on the hand, a hug, stroking the hair, a kiss on the cheek, a pat on the back. Gentle touch can be so reassuring.

12. Encourage your client to tell his stories on tape or in writing. This is an excellent opportunity for conversation about life stories and for a new life skill in memoir writing.

13. Seek help from other agencies, family members, a social worker, a volunteer, a nurse, the doctor, a chaplain or spiritual advisor. These resources might help you better understand your patient.

14. Positive communication is a great aid in helping your client deal with his fears or concerns. It also helps provide your patient with information about his/her condition. The unknown is always more frightening than dealing with reality. Remember: Some patients want to know everything and all at once. Others prefer that information come in parts. Look for clues to what your client wants to deal with.

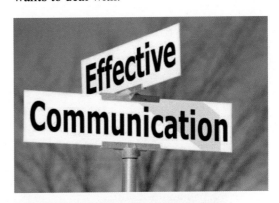

Chapter Six: Ethics, Integrity and Professional Behavior

One person caring about another represents

life's greatest value.

~Jim Rohn

What is a Code of Ethics?

Every profession has a code of ethics. This chapter outlines the basic principles and regulations essential to caregiving. Infractions could get you sued and/or result in the loss of your status as a certified caregiver.

Why Have a Code of Conduct?

Rules of Ethics are specific statements outlining what is considered the minimum level of acceptable professional conduct.

A code of conduct for a profession assures the public, and in particular those patients who will be cared for by caregivers, that they have a right to expect a specific level of behavior from caregivers. Moreover, if this level of care is not provided, they have actions they can take.

Caregivers as well as other healthcare professionals recognize and acknowledge that we are a diverse society. In their care, they embrace a multi-cultural approach to dealing with their clients. They pledge to support the worth, dignity, ability and uniqueness of their clients.

Caregivers have an official or unwritten Code of Ethics. They understand and acknowledge the vulnerability of the clients they serve and commit to provide highest possible standards of practice.

Accountability to Clients

A written or unwritten Code of Ethics creates a uniform standard to which caregivers will adhere. Having a code of ethics defines for both clients and the general public caregiver behavior. It outlines ethical responsibilities expected of caregivers and the organization for whom they work.

Education of Caregiver Professionals

A code of ethics acknowledges that caregivers come to their job with a wide variety of skills, knowledge, training and education. The code serves as a guide for both caregivers and their clients about the role and expectations of caregivers. The code describes the core values and principles of professional caregivers. These professionals are expected to understand and act in a manner consistent with their Code of Ethics.

Resolving Ethical Issues

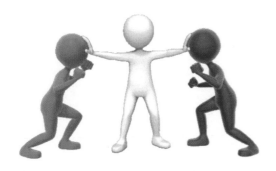

Not only does a Code of Ethics describe how caregivers are to behave. It also provides a framework for resolving issues where the actions of the caregiver are in question.

The code examines ethical dilemmas in all facets of a caregiver's work. It identifies the principles that need to be considered and what changes need to occur so conduct is in line with code of conduct.

Review of Complaints

Most codes of conduct have a process for reviewing complaints lodged by clients, their families, or caregivers themselves. These vary from state to state, province to province and country to country. Peer review may be part of this process.

The review process is the basis for assessing the merit of complaints and for resolving complaints against caregivers' practices.

Integrity

Caregivers are expected to honest, diligent, and accountable in the service they give their clients. They are expected to be consistent and punctual as well as professional in their appearance and service.

Loyalty and Responsibility

It is anticipated when you hire a caregiver that he/she will be trustworthy and dependable in service and relationships. A professional caregiver maintains client confidentiality, avoids conflicts of interest between client and other service providers, and acts at all times in the best interest of those he/she serves.

Enhancing Patient Benefits

A caregiver professional promotes clients' interests, values, and welfare. He/she provides service which enhances client benefits and avoids patient harm. A professional caregiver is always aware of the fact that conflicts that could arise. He/she considers the potential risk of interventions and strives for the well-being of clients at all times.

Clients' Rights and Dignity

A professional caregiver respects patient rights and aims to provide service that gives client dignity while maintaining patient privacy. He/she works to balance patient confidentiality with providing essential services.

Justice

The ideal caregiver treats patients fairly in all relationships. He/she avoids discrimination based on age, race, medical condition, ethnicity, gender, religion, sexual orientation, origin, disability, or socioeconomic level.

Patient/Caregiver Relationship

The ideal caregiver is a primary provider of service. While the referral may not come directly from the patient, the caregiver recognizes direct responsibility to his patient. All others related to this client are indirectly associated to the caregiver/client bond. These may include: relatives of the patient, other service professionals, community organizations, volunteers, money managers, neighbors, or friends. In the event of conflict needs, the requirements of the client will always come first.

Whether officially required, or professionally mandated, a professional caregiver will adhere to these ethical guidelines:

1. I will always treat my clients with kindness and respect.
2. I will always arrive at the client's home on time, preferably 5 minutes before the start of my scheduled hours. If I might be late, I will immediately call.
3. I will follow the Plan of Care each day for my client.
4. I will maintain a clean and organized home for my client.
5. I will never leave my client unattended. If the relief caregiver is late I will immediately call the Care Manager.
6. I will address my client by Mr or Ms, followed by their last name unless they invite me to use their first name.
7. I will honor the client's right to privacy and confidentiality, including their identity, address, and telephone number.
8. I will keep my religious beliefs, political choices, or personal issues within professional privacy and likewise respect my client's beliefs.
9. I will call 911 immediately when there is a medical emergency and then call my senior care company office or Care Manager.
10. I will not engage in financial transactions nor intimate

relationships with a client or family member.

11. I will never use alcohol or illegal drugs as a professional caregiver.

12. I will only use my personal mobile phone for calls and texts during rest or break periods.

Source: ***Professional Association of Caregivers Code of Ethics***

Chapter Seven: Cultural Sensitivity

"Impossible situations can become possible miracles."

–Robert H. Schuller

In North America, we live in a multicultural society. Between 2000 and 2010, USA saw a sharp increase in Asian immigrants. An even bigger influx of Hispanics was experienced in the same time period. While Hispanic immigrants increased by nearly 40%, non-Hispanic white immigrants increased by only 2%. Today, minorities outnumber whites in many communities in North America. This has resulted in a huge change in expectations about medical services as well as a sharp change in what is required of medical professionals.

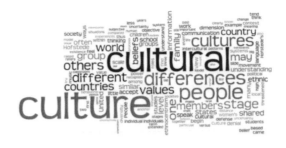

When caregivers find themselves working in a cross-cultural environment, it is crucial to have an understanding of the home and/or neighborhood. Otherwise, you may find yourself working in conflict with the beliefs and traditions of your client and his family or community. The ability to work with your patient and help him heal is contingent on your ability to communicate with the client and support him in rehabilitation. Culture plays a major role in defining the patient's understanding and responses to health care. Cultural ethics are a vital part of all aspects of medical care. Culture impacts a patient's understanding of his ailment and his willingness to accept health care.

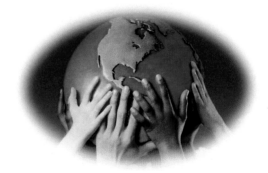

If healthcare professionals fail to understand the role culture plays in healing then they do not respect different cultures in providing health care. This lack of concern for understanding of culture may be a major detraction in patient rehabilitation.

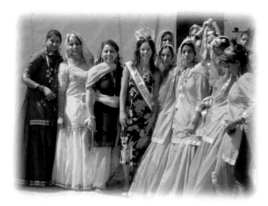

Cultural sensitivity is being aware as a caregiver that cultural differences and similarities between people exist. The ideal caregiver, while being aware of different cultures, assigns no one culture a positive or negative, better or worse, right or wrong value. The caregiver is aware that people are different but recognizes no one culture is superior.

Why is culture a concern?

Culture has a drastic effect on medical care. Culture affects people's decisions about illness, death, beliefs about treatment, and decisions about follow-up care. It affects how illness and pain are expressed, where and if patients seek help and preferred follow up treatment and care.

A healthcare professional knows that patient-caregiver communication can be improved and patient care can be enhanced if healthcare professionals can acknowledge and bridge the gap between medicine and the patient's beliefs and values and practices.

The ideal caregiver is aware of differences in ethnicity, heritage, nationality, age, religion, sexual orientation, disability, and socioeconomic status.

Caregivers can maximize this potential by learning more about patient's culture and yet focusing on the quality of patient care irrespective of cultural differences.

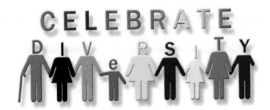

Cultural issues often affect patient expectations and interaction between the caregiver, the client's family and the client's cultural group. When the caregiver understands the cultural context of his/her patient's behavior, he/she can improve patient communication and service.

When a patient's culture clashes with the prevailing medical community, the patient's culture will generally prevail. This can cause problems in caregiver delivery of services as well as caregiver–patient relationships.

Caregivers can minimize the conflicting beliefs by increasing their understanding and awareness of the patient's culture and by being open minded and learning as much as possible about the client's culture.

Cultural competency, cultural awareness, or cultural sensitivity, can be defined as, an understanding and people skills that let

healthcare providers to recognize, appreciate, and operate inside an individual's cultural differences.

Ideal caregivers are aware of and accept patient's cultural differences and how these affect his adaptation to his care. When we as caregivers acknowledge our own cultural biases, we are a long way toward an awareness of how our culture differs from our patient's. When we acknowledge, and demonstrate our knowledge of these cultural differences, we promote trust and acceptance by our clients. This leads to better health care and higher acceptance of treatment.

Many cultural groups receive no medical care. Many of them are sadly underserved. There are many reasons for this. Caregivers need to be sensitive to the needs of each individual and how this fits into his/her beliefs, values, and perceptions.

One helpful idea is to determine whether a particular culture is collectivistic or individualistic. This information can help healthcare workers diagnose and plan for patient care. The following are examples of collectivistic cultural groups:

How does culture affect medical services?

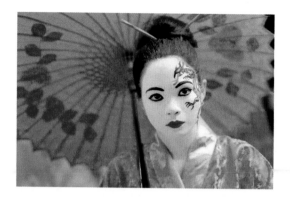

Take the **Amish** for example. They do not have health insurance. In general, Amish caregivers come from within their community and extended family. They expect that family and the Amish community will play an active role in nursing the sick, providing hospice for the dying and supporting the grieving family.

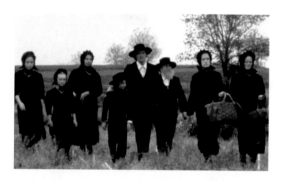

In the **Japanese** culture, supporting the sick psychologically and physically, by family and others is a way to motivate the patient to recover quickly. Historically, the Japanese have fought institutional health care. Institutions are in contravention of the Japanese respect for family members. Families will continue to care for members during hospitalization and take terminal members home to die.

In **Hispanic** families, it is expected that family members would be involved in medical decisions such as the need for surgery. The doctor would explain the need to the entire family before the patient signed consent forms.

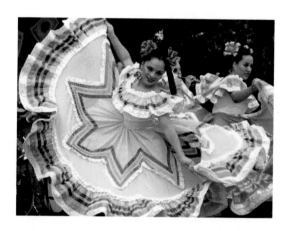

When cultural or language differences complicate it just think how scary it is. Medicine in North America has developed into a unique subculture with its own language, behaviors, expectations, strategies, technologies, and problems. Health care then transects two boundaries for those from different cultures.

Cross-cultural circumstances often magnify the space between the views of patients and healthcare professionals.

Professionals must employ approaches that recognize discrepancy in views and values of the individual, his culture and the medical professional.

When the caregiver associates with the client, their dialogue requires a lot more than sounds. There is socialization. The medical professional makes observations and, through questioning, he arrives at a diagnosis, or changes in that diagnosis. Planning, sharing, and negotiation ensues. During this verb interchange, the caregiver can assess the plan and needed changes. Cultural differences often present language and/or ideological barriers to comprehension or even resistance to the proposed plan. Patient and caregiver may be at odds about goals of the caregiver program, the type of therapy and even the patient's contribution to his therapy. Indeed, there may be a wide—and undiscovered— discrepancy between the views of patient and caregiver about what are realistic expectations.

Chapter Eight: Appearance and Hygiene

Life's challenges are not supposed to paralyze you; they're supposed to help you discover who you are.

~Bernice Johnson Reagon

Because you are a healthcare professional there are certain expectations about your attire and grooming.

Hygiene

Caregivers are expected to meet certain minimum hygiene requirements while they are at work. These include:

- General cleanliness by bathing daily.
- Regular oral hygiene three times a day brushing and flossing of teeth.
- Applying deodorant or anti-perspirant to minimize body odors.
- Avoidance of heavily scented perfumes, colognes, sprays and/or lotions. To mitigate patient and/or co-worker allergic reactions, migraines and respiratory difficulties.
- Nails clean and trimmed under a quarter inch in length.
- Regular hand wash and disinfecting after eating, or using the washroom.

Personal Grooming

- Uniform or other required clothing clean, pressed, appropriately fitted and in good repair.
- Socks or hose worn with shoes.

- Hair tidy and well-groomed hair. Sideburns, mustaches and beards trimmed. No unnatural hair colors deemed unprofessional.

- Long hair tied back to avoid being caught in equipment.

- Moderate make-up.

- Clothing fitted so it does not get caught in equipment.

- No dark glasses unless prescribed by an optical specialist.

- Avoidance of dangling or large hoop jewelry that could constitute a safety risk. If a pencil can be passed through a hoop earring it is not safe to wear while operating equipment.

- Body piercing limited to three per ear. Any additional visible body piercing is unacceptable.

- Offensive, hostile, and/or unprofessional tattoos that are visible while working are forbidden.

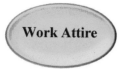

Work Attire

At all times, caregivers should adhere to the dress code of the organization. If you are a self-employed caregiver, wear appropriate scrubs that looks professional and allows you to move about freely to do your job.

Unless stated otherwise the following should be considered inappropriate attire:

- Sweat pants, yoga pants, jogging pants, gym shorts, bicycle shorts, athletic shorts

- Pants that expose midriff, underwear, butt crack

- Low-cut tops, halter tops, tops with spaghetti straps

- Tops that expose the midriff or underwear;

- Mini-skirts;

- See through, mesh, opaque clothing

- Clothing that is offensive, controversial, distracting, and/or disruptive

- Clothing that is overtly commercial, has a political, personal or offensive message

- Plastic flip-flops, sandals, beach footwear, high heeled shoes, open-toed shoes that pose a safety risk.

Personal Protective Equipment

Caregivers are expected to use prescriber protective safety equipment at all times in areas where required. Depending on the type of clients caregivers are serving, the following personal protective equipment may at times—or all the time—be required.

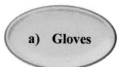

a) Gloves

If you are handling blood-soiled items, bodily fluids, excretions, wound secretions and/or surfaces contaminated by the above materials, always wear gloves.

Gloves should also be worn if in doubt of any substance. Be sure gloves fit.

If performing a clinical procedure always wear disposable gloves. If the procedure requires sterile procedure like cleaning a wound, always wear sterile gloves. If you have cuts, scratches, or lesions, always wear gloves. If a glove is torn during a procedure, remove it and replace it immediately. Change gloves after contact with any infected material. Discard used gloves before leaving patient's room. Wash and disinfect hands immediately after discarding gloves. Remove gloves by pinching glove at wrist. Pull glove toward fingertip turning it inside out. Ball up and discard. Repeat process with other glove.

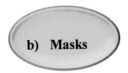

Masks should be worn to protect the caregiver from inhaling microorganisms. Disposable masks should be worn whenever there is a perceived danger of infection. Properly applied, a mask fits snugly over mouth, nose, and chin so infectious organisms cannot enter or escape. The top edge should fit below protective glasses. Keep talking to a minimum while wearing the mask. Discard mask if it becomes damp. Remove gloves before removing mask. Dispose of mask after each use. Wash hands after removing mask.

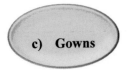

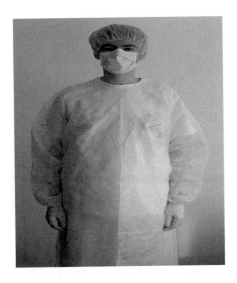

Wear an apron or gown to protect clothing from being soiled during a procedure. Use a sterile gown if performing a sterile procedure. Ensure gown or apron is made of moisture resistant material. Change gown after procedure. Place in the appropriate receptacle for destruction.

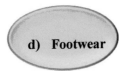

It is vital that caregiver shoes provide support, grip, and fit well. Slides and flip flops and those trendy stilettos do not provide a firm footing if you are lifting, bending and/or pulling. You need a shoe that provides more support and stability than ballet flats or clogs. If your shoes are too large you may trip. They won't support those hours on your feet. Easy to access shoes like flip flops, slides, mules, clogs, slippers, sandals are potentially hazardous at work. They can slip off endangering the client and the caregiver. You can trip in them and they do not provide stability or support for those long days spent on your feet. If your foot is unsupported it can turn inward or outward, causing permanent damage to your instep or sole.

On the other hand, tight-fitting footwear or footwear that offers too much grip can also cause injuries or painful bone deformities. Special duty shoes with reinforced toes and ones that allow added orthotics will offer support for such ailments as weak or fallen arches, sensitive soles, hammertoes, bunions or any other ailment which standing on your feet causes.

Walking/ running shoes come in a wide range designs. They are available at affordable prices. They are durable and available in various weights, soles and toe/heel box configurations. Most can also be washed and dried.

Running shoes can be laced up or have Velcro closures for easy on/off. Be good to your feet with proper shoes and good foot care. Clip toenails. Moisturize feet. Watch out for ailments like toenail fungus, athlete's foot, corns, bunions and warts. Try a regular footbath. Use clean socks every day and add

a thin coat of lotion or Vaseline to top and bottom of feet.

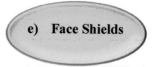

e) Face Shields

Equipment like goggles and face shields are worn to prevent body fluids from getting into the caregiver's eyes. While this is not always necessary, if body fluids are involved in the caregiving, face shields are a good precautionary measure.

f) Goggles

Wearing goggles ensures that flying materials do not injure the caregiver's eyes. Goggles also prevent contact with germs.

g) Respirator

In rare situations, a caregiver might be exposed to airborne dangers. Such situations would include things like tuberculosis or chicken pox. In situations like this, caregivers should wear a gown, gloves, and a respirator. Illnesses that travel long distances through the air are usually handled in hospital quarantine settings but before the disease is diagnosed, caregivers could be exposed.

It's important to have all safety equipment available and to know which you need to use in each case. All the above equipment is not necessary in every patient-care situation. Which is needed depends on what type of germ, bacteria, or infection you may be exposed to. For example, when dealing with certain types of infections or matter, you may need a mask or goggles or a face shield. Other situations may require only a gown and/or gloves. When making a choice, err on the side of being over-protected.

Keep in mind, there is a standard precaution when you are working with all clients—no matter what the situation. Any time you are handling blood or urine or fecal matter or other body fluids it is necessary for your personal safety to wear gloves, a mask and gown as a bare minimum.

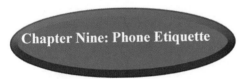

Chapter Nine: Phone Etiquette

Too often we underestimate the power of a

touch, a smile, a kind word, a listening ear,

an honest compliment, or the smallest act of

caring, all of which have the potential to

turn a life around.

~Leo Buscaglia

WHAT IS TELEPHONE ETIQUETTE?

Telephone etiquette involves the proper way to answer the phone, make calls, leave messages, return calls, and deal with difficult callers.

Why is phone etiquette Important?

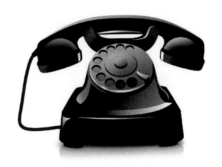

Knowing and employing good telephone etiquette is part of your professional duties as a caregiver. When you fail to use proper phone etiquette, you leave a bad impression of you as a professional, your patient, and the agency or department for which you work.

When you use good phone etiquette, callers are left with a favorable impression of you, your employer, your profession and your client. If you are an independent caregiver, how you make and receive calls might make or break your business. You and those you employ who answer your business phone are ambassadors of your profession and your business.

Key Things to Remember about Phone Etiquette

- Use those company manners your mother taught you. Say, "Thank you" and "Please." Call people by name.

- Maintain a professional demeanor. You are not talking to a friend. This is business.

- Listen carefully. Take notes to be sure you got the message correctly

- Avoid interrupting.

- Make follow-up comments or ask follow-up questions to clarify.

- Be invitational. I once had a secretary who should never have answered the phone. She made every caller dread having to call my department.

- Don't ignore the phone's ringing and make people wait or leave messages.

- If you MUST have one of those irritating automated answering systems, make it simple and invitational.

- When you call, make it clear who you are, in what capacity you are calling and to whom you want to speak.

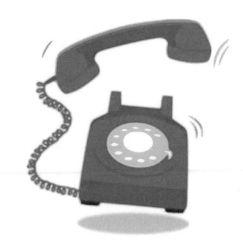

When Answering Calls

- Answer promptly. Identify yourself and the business or household.

- Don't rush your caller response. Give the caller time to process what you've said.

- Be friendly and professional.

- Ask how you may help or to whom you may direct the call.

- Smile. The caller cannot see you but your smile telegraphs in your voice.

- Speak clearly in a pleasant "announcer style" voice.

- Ask for the caller's name. Note it and the time of the call.

- Ask to whom the caller wishes to speak. Direct the call efficiently.

- If it is a wrong number, be polite. If it is possible to redirect the call to the correct receiver, do so efficiently and courteously.

- If you have to redirect the call, use the hold button so the caller is not privy to background conversations.

- Use a message pickup or answering machine service if you can't be near the phone to take calls.

- Return calls as soon as possible.

When Making Calls

- **Identify yourself and your organization or affiliation. If you are calling about a specific client give that information as well**

- **State your purpose for calling.**

- **If you reach a wrong number, apologize and hang up.**

- **If you agreed to call at a specific time, do so.**

- **If you have to reschedule a call, let the receiver know why and set another time to call back.**

- **Leave a message clearly identifying yourself, your affiliation and the reason for the call. Be sure to leave a contact number. Ask for a return call or tell the receiver when you will call back.**

Dealing with Rude or Irritating Callers

- Be polite and diplomatic.

- Don't get rude, angry or confrontational.

- If it's a telemarketer or other unsolicited call, be polite but firm. "I'm sorry. We're not interested."

- If the caller is phoning about a misunderstanding or problem, listen politely without interrupting.

- Demonstrate willingness to resolve the situation, problem or misunderstanding.

- Put yourself in the caller's shoes. If the family member or member of the caregiver team or neighbor is angry or frustrated, impatient or upset, think about why this is so and empathize.

- Show a willingness to assist the caller in addressing concerns.

- Offer to have someone higher up in the supervisory chain call the person back.

- If the call is for your patient and it isn't a convenient time, say so and suggest calling back at a time that is better or take a message.

- If it is a confrontational call, be calm, polite but firm. Speak slowly and clearly.

- **Putting the Caller on Hold**

  - Know how to use the hold feature on your phone's system and use it.

  - Use the hold feature so the caller doesn't overhear background noise/conversations.

  - When putting a caller on hold, ask permission. "May I put you on hold for a minute?" Tell the caller you are going to put him/her on hold and do so for only a short period. Then get back to him promptly.

  - If other lines are ringing, write line # and caller's name before saying, "Hold please."

Then when you get back to the caller, you can call him by name.

- **Transferring Calls**
  - • Ask the caller to whom you may direct his call. Transfer it to that line rather than giving him an extension # so he does not have to call again. This saves him time, inconvenience and perhaps cost if he is calling long distance.
  - • Stay on the line to make sure the call was transferred properly.
  - • If you are transferring the call, tell him to who, you are transferring him.
  - • If that person is unavailable transfer him to the receiver's voice mail.

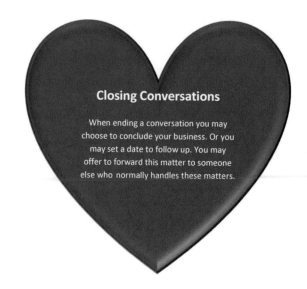

Closing Conversations

When ending a conversation you may choose to conclude your business. Or you may set a date to follow up. You may offer to forward this matter to someone else who normally handles these matters.

How to Take Messages

- Have pen and paper ready.

- Take the message and read it back to the caller to be certain you have it right.

- Make sure you have the caller's name spelled correctly.

- Be certain you have taken the phone # correctly.

- Be as detailed and specific about the reason for the call as you can.

- Be sure to add: date, time, of the call and your name.

- Place the message where the receiver will see it right away.

- Offer to transfer caller to voice mail instead of taking a message.

Try to resolve the issue or at least take it to the next step.

Try to end on a positive note. You might try one or more of these strategies on a call that has gone on too long and clearly will not end in resolution

- Apologize for not being able to resolve the issue.

- Offer to finish the conversation at a later date.

- End on a positive note.

- Say you've enjoyed the discussion

- Ask clarifying questions.

- Aim for a pleasant closing such as: "Have a nice day." or "It was nice talking to you."

Be honest. If you cannot help, commiserate but don't make false promises or attempt to scapegoat.

Always be polite.

Don't get into a verbal battle with the caller.

If the caller becomes abusive, tell him you will have your supervisor talk to the caller.

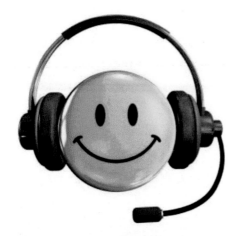

Using Voice Mail Effectively

Voice mail has many benefits and advantages when used properly. However, there are also some things to consider.

Some people do not like to leave or receive voice mail. Know when this is the case and don't offer it as an option.

If you have agreed to receive voice mail, listen to it and respond in a timely fashion.

Always offer voice mail as an option instead of taking a written message unless you know the caller or receiver do not like this option.

Creating a Voice Mail Salutation

Avoid cutsie or racy salutations. Be professional.

Tell whose voice mail it is. For example: "Hello, you've reached the voice mail of_____at_____."

Give the date.

Avoid salutations like, "Good morning" or "Good afternoon". They will bed wrong half the time. Instead, say, "Good day" or "Hello."

Tell why you are unable to take the call and when you will be back at your desk.

Record your own message. Avoid "canned" messages.

Try to make the message welcoming and personal.

Leave an alternative in case the caller needs to talk instead to someone else in your department. Offer instructions for talking to someone else like dialing an extension or pressing zero.

Keep your greeting as short and uncomplicated as you can.

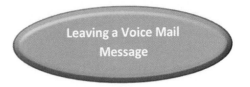

Leaving a Voice Mail Message

Just as there is etiquette to creating a voice mail salutation, there are tips about leaving a good voice mail message.

Identify yourself, your organization and your department

Tell the receiver what you are calling about

Leave a number where you can be reached.

Speak clearly and slowly. Don't mumble.

Try to call from a location where background noise is not an issue.

At the end of your call, remind the receiver who you are and repeat your phone contact information.

End on a polite note like, "Have a great day." Or "Looking forward to receiving your call."

Avoid distractions like chewing gum, smoking, drinking a beverage, or eating while answering a call or making one. Call from a location free of traffic, background voices, machines… if at all possible. Avoid using poor grammar, slang, profanity or other non-standard speech.

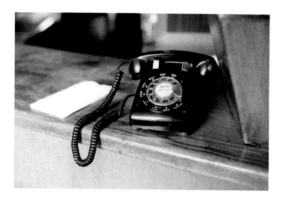

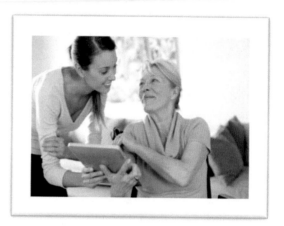

Checking Messages and Returning Calls

If you are accepting voice mail and/or someone is taking messages for you then the caller has every right to expect a timely return call.

> Check voice mail/written messages regularly throughout the day and return calls as soon as possible. Within twenty-four hours is a reasonable call back expectation.

Chapter Ten: Escorting and Transporting your Patient

Compassion automatically invites you to relate with people because you no longer regard people as a drain on your energy."

~ Chogyam Trungpa

Reason for Transport

Your patient may require transport for

several reasons. He/she may have

Telephone may be the first exposure someone has to you and your profession. We all know how important first impressions are. Keep your voice loud enough to hear but not unpleasantly loud, pleasant, clear and a nice tone.

experienced a fall or deterioration of health or an illness. If you are a caregiver who works independently or for a caregiver agency, part of your stated responsibilities may include transporting your client to appointments, doing errands, shopping, attending social functions.

If this is the case, you may be asked to provide a car and drive it or you may be asked to drive a vehicle available to the client. In either case there are liability issues. Consider these scenarios:

You assume your car insurance covers passengers transported as part of your job.

This is certainly an issue you should be raising with your insurance company and with the people who employ you. NEVER assume your automotive insurance covers this scenario.

If you are to transport clients to get groceries, run errands or attend medical appointments, and the client and/or company you work for expects you to use your personal vehicle, make sure you have liabilities covered by your insurance and/or company insurance. Get written documentation and put it with your insurance information. Keep duplicates of both the letter and your insurance policy in a file that is not in your car.

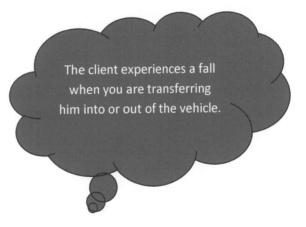

The client experiences a fall when you are transferring him into or out of the vehicle.

As long as you are transferring your client in a safe and established manner, you have nothing to fear ethically, legally, or professionally. However, falls are unsettling for both caregiver and client. Discuss improved transfer strategies so this does not recur.

insurance company that you have their permission to transport your client.

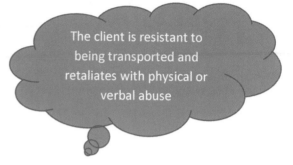

Your first priority should always be the safety of your client. If you have any doubts about his well-being insist he be transported to hospital for checking his health. Inform the family of the incident and your actions.

You should have done your research regarding patient transport before you ever put a client in your vehicle. If you have, you should also have a letter from your insurance company stating that they are aware of your occasional use of your vehicle to transport clients and that you are covered by your insurance for these instances. Report the accident in the same way you would report any accident. Remind your

This is an issue like all other issues of patient resistance. Treat the outburst the same way you would in the home. You can be diplomatic. You can be persuasive. You cannot physically force your client to get into that vehicle. Try to get at the reason your client refuses to co-operate. Take note of the incident and report it and the outcome to your supervisor and to the designated family member. If there might be a solution, suggest it to them.

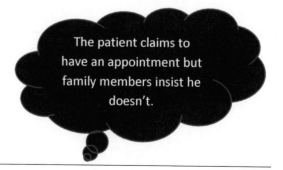

Your client may be confused. Your client could also be using this excuse to get out of the house because he is bored or resistant to rules. On the other hand, perhaps the family is uninformed. Try to check on the validity of his claim and resolve the issue to everyone's satisfaction.

The vehicle you've been asked to use for transport is not suitable for moving this client.

Your first priority is your client's safety. If the vehicle is unsafe for patient transfer, speak to whoever is requesting you to perform this duty and state that it is unsafe to do so. Explain why and suggest an alternative vehicle. Make notes about the issue and date them. Perhaps the vehicle no longer constitutes a safe transport for your client and it is time for the decision makers to think about using a mobility vehicle service.

You sustain extra costs for vehicle insurance, fuel, and maintenance due to transporting a client

This is an issue on which you need to be clear at the beginning of your employment. If you agreed to transport and did not get clarification when you accepted the job then you have little recourse except to reopen a discussion. Keep records of costs of insurance, fuel, vehicle maintenance, licensing and a log of the miles you drive patient. Discuss these costs with your employer.

Before you begin a job, ask questions about your responsibilities—including transportation.

Your agency has assigned you a client. Caregiver duties according to this agency, do not include transportation. The client and her family request that you transport her to .

If your duties do not include transportation, you need to make this clear at the initial meeting and again when it comes up. If necessary, have the agency provide written and oral corroboration of your no-transport stand. There are many agencies whose rule is: Never under any circumstances take any client or family member in your vehicle while working on contract for them.

Because your agency has a no transport rule the client and family have asked you to accompany your client to appointments and social functions on public transportation.

Remember: Your priority is your client's safety. If the vehicle is unsafe for patient transfer, speak to whoever is requesting you to perform this duty and state that it is unsafe to do so and why. Suggest a safer mode of transportation than public transportation such as an accessible taxi service or a mobility bus.

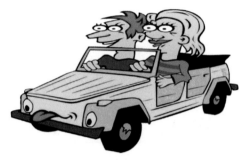

You've been asked to accompany your client while a friend or family member drives the vehicle.

You can travel with the patient in a car that is driven by a family member, or taxi in most cases. This needs to be clarified by your agency. Remember: Your first priority is your client's safety. If the vehicle and/or the driver is/are unsafe for patient transfer in your professional opinion, speak to whoever is requesting you to perform this duty and state that it is unsafe to do so and why. Suggest a safer mode of transportation than a family car such as an accessible taxi service or a mobility bus.

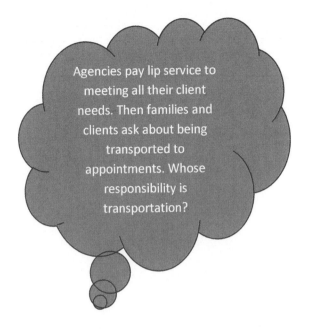

You've been asked to accompany your client in a taxi to appointments or social functions.

You can travel with the patient in a taxi in most cases. However, be sure to clarify this with your agency.

Remember: Your first priority is your client's safety. If the mode of transportation is unsafe for patient transfer, in your professional opinion, speak to whoever is requesting you to travel by taxi. State that it is unsafe to do so and why. Suggest a safer

mode of transportation such as an accessible taxi vehicle or a mobility bus.

Agencies pay lip service to meeting all their client needs. Then families and clients ask about being transported to appointments. Whose responsibility is transportation?

Unless specifically spelled out, caregivers are not medical personnel. Unless medical personnel like ambulance workers are tasked with medical or emergency transport, they do not provide transportation. If non-emergency transport is provided as part of a caregiver service, most agencies have the client or his/her designate sign a waiver that protects you, the caregiver, and the agency, should something happen when you are providing transport. It's the same kind of waiver that protects volunteer drivers for Cancer Society or Meals on Wheels or

Children's Aid Society drivers who transport District Child Services wards.

However, remember this about waivers: We live in a society that looks for ways to sue. Even if waivers are signed, these may not stand up in court. Even if they do, you may still incur legal costs for the case to go to court. Bottom line? Even if you are being paid, err on the side of patient safety and your peace of mind and suggest accessible transportation.

Whether you are responsible to provide transportation or even act as a companion to appointments and social events, it should be clearly spelled out in your job description. The kind of reimbursement you are given should also be clearly stated on your written contract. If no mention is made about providing transportation and/or companion services in transit, ask that it be clearly stated in your contract.

Don't take this duty upon yourself unless it is stated clearly in writing that it is an expected duty. It is way too risky. You are a caregiver, not a taxi service.

There are safe alternatives for transportation of patients and these services are insured.

Chapter Eleven: Caregiver Observation Skills:

As a primary caregiver you are in a position to note changes in your patient's behavior, habits, and personality. You can be a big help to the medical professionals in observing things that have changed.

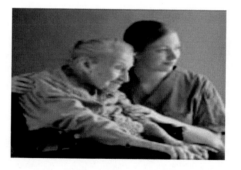

Deciding what kind of support your client needs is a matter of dialogue with your client, his family and sometimes other medical support personnel. Having a family meeting is a good opportunity to discuss care needs and aid in the decision-making process. Consider the type of help with dressing, bathing, lifting, medication management, companionship, housekeeping, and/or transportation your client needs.

Find out what family member(s) are in charge of caregiving and/or care arrangement.Learn what days and times your client needs assistance. Can you handle this level of assistance or will the family need to apply for added services? What types of help are the client's friends and family members able and prepared to provide?

Having gotten a picture of the client's caregiver needs and any out-of-home assistance liked physiotherapy he needs and must be transported to, you are then in a better situation to care for and provide observations

Observation plays a key role in diagnosis and treatment of a client. An experienced eye for observation provides clues to when something is a medical emergency and knowing who to contact. Each client is different. Therefore, approaches will also vary. It is important that the caregiver notes changes and keep detailed records.

The following are observation skills and strategies:

Observe and Establish Normal Baseline for your Client

Your first task will be to establish a baseline. What is normal for this patient. You can do this through early observations, medical reports, dialogue with the client and/or his family. This establishes the base upon which you can make observations of changes in behavior, medical stats, and/or attitude.

Compare Subsequent Observations to Previous Baseline

Once this baseline is established, you as a healthcare professional can noted any improvements and/or deterioration in your client's condition.

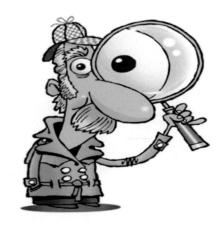

Look for Changes In Breathing, Fever, Cough, Chills, Chest Pain

Many of these changes you can note through observation and/or taking temperature.

- **Note Nausea/Vomiting, Unusual Thirst, Change In Skin Color**

These may be signs of a medical emergency.

Look for Changes in Output, Color and/or Odor Frequency, Sediment of Urine

Changes in urine may signal an infection, kidney problem or even detect another disease like sugar in the urine would detect diabetes.

- **Document Patient's Level of Alertness, Mood and/or Behavior**

Changes in behavior/attitude may signal medical problems.

- **Check Dehydration or Edema**

Both are signs of circulation problems that might flag other conditions.

- **Note Changes In Appetite, Eating Habits, And Bowel Changes**

Changes in these activities may be medical signals the body is giving.

- Observe Changes In Level Of Functional Abilities

Is your client less able to move, complete activities he could do at the baseline assessment.

- Reporting
The ability to take detailed and accurate notes on observations is vital.

- **Deviations In Client Conditions That Must Be Reported Immediately/Later**
Reporting deviations after recording is crucial to avoiding what could become a medical emergency.

- **How To Report Observations, Who To Report Observations To**

It is important that protocol for sharing observations be set up at the outset with your patient and his family so there is no confusion.

Recording a Proper Documentation Using Common Medical Terminology

Learning to record observations so everyone knows and understands them is important. There are courses for caregivers who wish to hone their observation and recording skills. Early detection can often save a patient's life if it is documented accurately and shared in a timely fashion.

Chapter Twelve: Handling Medical Emergencies

"You gain strength, courage, and confidence by every experience in which you really stop to look fear in the face. You must do the things which you think you cannot do."

~ Eleanor Roosevelt

The fact that you as a caregiver will have to deal with medical emergencies is a likelihood. One in three seniors suffers a fall that requires emergency assistance each year. It's important to know when a situation is an emergency and to know what to do.

Your patients are often at higher risk because of age, frailty, Alzheimer's, heart disease, diabetes or other medical conditions.

It's important for both you and your client to remain calm.

BE PREPARED

If you are prepared for an emergency, your reaction isn't to panic. How can you be prepared? Make a list of important facts about your patient. Update it regularly. Put it somewhere easy to grab. Make a second copy for your car. Include:

Client's full name

- Date of birth

- Social Security number

- Insurance information

- Medications and dosages

- Doctors, dates of last visit, test results

- Brief medical history listing medical conditions

Keep a current list of phone numbers of those to contact in an emergency.

Contact Your Local EMS

EMS should have an address on file.

Learn First Aid

Get training in first aid and CPR. Make sure it is up to date. Keep a stocked first aid kit.

Pack Your Bags

Keep an overnight bag packed with a two-day supply of medications, pajamas, toothbrush and toiletries. Have a bag for yourself in case you end up staying at the hospital. Include books, snacks, a change of clothing and emergency phone numbers.

If emergencies are prepared for and you treat them as a process—not a crisis—you and your client will be better off.

Chapter Thirteen: Fire and Safety Preparedness

Be determined to handle any challenge in a way that will make you grow."

~Les Brown

As a caregiver, the responsibility for what to do in emergency situations falls on you. There are many ways to prepare for this eventuality. Organizations like the American Crisis Prevention & Management Association (ACPMA), National Caregiver Certification Association (NCCA). Within these courses you can learn the five basic fire safety practices required in a healthcare setting.

Your patients are among the most vulnerable during a crisis. Preparedness is key. The following suggestions are offered by California's firefighters:

Emergency Preparedness

1.   Develop a Communication Plan:

Know the people in the neighborhood. In the event of a disaster, check in on each other. Create a list of emergency contacts. Keep a copy near the phones and a copy in your wallet or purse.

2. Take Health Precautions:

List all your client's medical conditions. Encourage clients to have a medical ID bracelet. List patient's medications.

Store a two-week supply of medications in a safe, accessible place.

Look into community programs such as *File of Life* or *Vial of Life* to aid in medical information storage.

3. Plan for Evacuation:

Evacuate immediately upon notification.

Have a vehicle available for evacuation. Know evacuation routes. Always keep vehicle gassed up or charged just in case. Drive the evacuation route just so you know it.Check where to obtain an emergency supply of medication or emergency medical care in case of a disaster.

4. Prepare an Evacuation Kit:

Keep a two-week supply of medication on hand in its original packaging. List all medications your client is taking (both over-the-counter and prescription).

Get from your client's doctor a note documenting medical conditions and how they are treated. Keep it and two-week supply in evacuation kit. If your client requires medical equipment pack duplicate equipment like: spare blood glucose monitoring system, blood pressure monitor, hearing aid batteries, or oxygen. Pack basic supplies: three-day food and water supply, maps, clothing, blankets, toiletries, cash, first aid kit.

Pack important documents: wills, deeds, bank account information and tax records.

Other items to add to your emergency kit: batteries, flashlights and a battery- operated radio, one blanket per person.

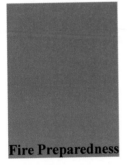 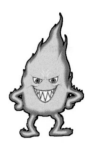

Fire Preparedness

Being prepared for fires is not difficult and it could very well save lives.

1. *Smoke Alarms:* *Make sure every bedroom, hallway, and kitchen has smoke alarms. Test these monthly and replace batteries in spring and fall.*

2. **Smell of Smoke***: If you smell smoke, gather patient, pets and any other occupants. Evacuate immediately. Call the 911 and yell fire at the top of your lungs to ensure the neighborhood knows.*

3. **Crawl on the Floor:** *Crawl to the nearest exit. Wet a washcloth to cover client's face and your own.*

4. **Check for Hot Doors:** *When you hear the smoke alarm or smell smoke, check the door before you open it. If it is hot the fire is just outside that door. Do not open the door. Break a window to get out.*

5. **Stop, Drop, and Roll.** *If fire has attacked your clothes, get outside immediately. Then stop, drop to the ground, and roll until the fire is out.*

6. **Home Fire Hazards:** *Matches, lighters, cigarettes, candles, curling irons, coffee pots, stoves, and fireplaces are often sources of fire if neglected. Make sure appliances are off and unplugged. Don't light candles or leave matches or lighters lying around.*

7. **Emergency Fire Preparedness:** *Being prepared for an emergency or disaster situation is one of the best things you can do to save your family from danger. Have an evacuation plan in case of fire. Practice it regularly.*

Chapter Fourteen: Proper Hygiene Assistance

Some days there won't be a song in your heart. Sing anyway."

~ Emory Austin

Attending to the hygiene needs of your client can be a sticky situation. Many patients are embarrassed to disrobe or toilet in front of others. Given their lack of mobility transfers can be physically demanding for the caregiver. However, there are ways to make the job easier and more comfortable for both patient and caregiver.

1. Create a comfortable environment.

While the task of helping a loved one bathe, dress, or toilet can be difficult for caregivers, they are even more stressful and embarrassing for your patient. That's why it is vital to create as peaceful a setting as you can. Quiet comfort relieves embarrassment and promotes well-being. Consider peaceful music, subdued lighting and even aromatherapy to soothe your client and distract from the job at hand.

2. Take Your Cue from Your Client

Many older adults hate change. Aim at keeping routines as close to normal as possible. Acknowledge your patient's needs, fears, and preferences. As much as possible—within safety guidelines—encourage your client to do as much as he can by himself. Keep to accepted hygiene standards. A senior may require a full bath or shower twice a week and sponge baths in between. He/she may be able to handle the sponge baths independently.

3. Encourage Independence

Patients involved in self-care facilitates continuing independence. Today there are lots of types of adaptive equipment to make bathing and grooming both easier and safer for aging hands.

Look into safety equipment for kitchen and bathroom. Grab bars, nonslip floor adhesives, raised toilets, support bars at toilet, tub and kitchen sink help seniors in the bathroom and kitchen carry out their life with minimal assistance and safety. Seek the advice of an occupational therapist for sound advice.

4. Minimize Client Discomfort

You can reduce the embarrassment and awkwardness of client personal care and hygiene tasks by pre-planning. Set water and room temperature at comfort level. Have a warm fluffy towel or robe ready. Make sure your conversations and your body language have no signs of stress, irritation, or embarrassment. This sets the\ tone for the task. The more comfortable you are the less your client will be uncomfortable.

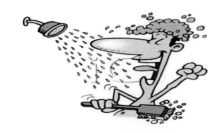

5. Make Use of Resources.

No matter what the relationship was between the parent and child—whatever it was—this is going to be extremely challenging because it is not logical. There's no way to deal with it rationally or directly. You don't reason it out. What I've said to so many people is: we always must lead with our love.

~ Dr. Stephen Hoag *A Son's Handbook: Bringing Up Mom with Alzheimer's/Dementia*

Millions of caregivers all over America have a wealth of information. Log onto chat lines. Read good resource materials. (See Helpful Resources section.) You may work alone but there are many resources at your fingertips.

Consider joining a local caregivers' support group. Benefit from the wealth of experience and knowledge out there. The more you learn about good practices and coping techniques, the more prepared you'll be to face tasks like making transfers, toileting, bathing and other personal hygiene with knowledge, confidence and poise.

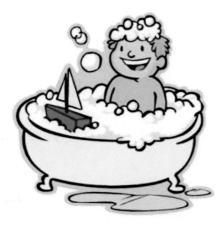

What Do Caregivers Want to See in Training?

Caregivers want a program that is practical and gives them hands-on training so they will be competent to deal with whatever arises. They want training that prepares them to take good care of their clients. They want to graduate from the caregiver program prepared, confident and ready to make their patients happy, well looked after and comfortable.

Caregivers do not want a theoretical program that makes them "book smart" but unprepared for the actualities of their job.

Caregivers want courses that are taught by actual practicing caregivers. They do not want to hear from those who have never actually fulfilled the caregiver role.

In this era of online training, it is helpful to back up your online training with watching videos to really see how things are done. Take advantage of training organizations like the National Caregiver Certification Association (NCCA). Their website is www.thencca.com

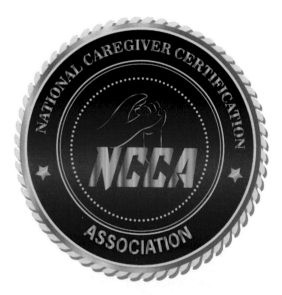

What do Clients Want Their Caregivers to Know?

Home Care Pulse conducted interviews with home care clients and their families to see what they most wanted their caregivers to know. Many of them expressed concern that their caregiver would know how to help them transfer safely. They wanted caregivers who were capable of assessing their needs

and creating a plan to meet those needs. They wanted caregivers who knew how to respond competently to emergency situations.

They wanted people who were trained and comfortable helping them with personal hygiene needs like bathing, hair washing, dressing, and toileting.

What Agencies who Hire Caregivers Want their Hirees to Know

When agencies consider hiring caregivers they are looking for competent, knowledgeable, able-bodied individuals who work well as part of a healthcare team.

They want caregivers who show initiative and have an understanding of the agency's rules. They want people who have good communication skills. They want employees with keen observation skills who take detailed notes and share their observations with all the stakeholders in their client's life.

They want enthusiastic, cheerful employees who are dedicated and responsible.

They want workers who are up to date on the latest strategies in caregiving and are prepared to continue to take upgrading courses to stay current in such areas as:

Patient Transfers

- Transferring clients using lifting techniques and lift technology including: Hoyer Lift and transfer boards.

Bathing

- Using proper techniques and helpful tips for bathing those with physical challenges.

Working with Memory Challenged Clients

- Characteristics of Alzheimer's and dementia
- Knowledge of how to work with clients who suffer from mental cognition issues. Understanding of symptoms of Alzheimer's and dementia
- Understanding of how to observe these symptoms.
- Strategies for providing consistent, reassuring, and compassionate care for the memory challenged.

Incontinence Care

- How to keep clients clean, dry and infection free.
- How to help clients retain their dignity in these embarrassing situations.

Colostomy and Catheter Training

- Knowledge of what they can and cannot do as caregivers.
- Training in caregiver care of these clients.

- Training in tasks such as proper/sanitary methods for emptying waste
- Understanding of and ability to keep clients clean, dry, and free of infections.

Patient Safety

- How to keep clients—and themselves—safe in all situations.
- On-the-job safety for caregivers
- In-the-home safety for clients.
- What to do in emergency situations.

Company Policies, Procedures and Goals

- A knowledge of what the agency expects of professional caregivers hired by your company.
- Employer expectations and your agency goals.

Homemaking Skills

- Ability to make simple meals
- Knowledge of how to shop
- Understanding of how to keep working environment clean and tidy
- Basic menu planning skills
- Ability to operate household appliances safely

Death and Dying

- Caregivers understanding of client's terminal illness
- Ability to work with those who are facing death
- Stamina to lose a client who has become a friend
- Training in how to assist a client or the family dealing with shock, grief or loss

Caregiver Certification

Look for a local caregiver school in your area to obtain certification. Alternatively, for a good online training, visit www.thencca.com

Useful resources

AgingCare.com. "How to Find and Manage Home Care". https://www.agingcare.com/ebook/home-care?ebs=rtfhg

Alzheimer's Association. "Take Care of Yourself".

http://www.alz.org/national/documents/brochure_caregiverstress.pdf

AlzOnline. "Dealing with Abuse, Neglect, Threats, or Other Selfish Use of others Receiving Care"
http://alzonline.phhp.ufl.edu/en/reading/abuse.php

Bayshore Healthcare. "Aging at Home"
https://www.bayshore.ca/aging-at-home/?gclid=CMXPsI_5o9MCFd26wAodr_cIQg

Boss, P. (2011) *Loving Someone who has Dementia*. *https://www.amazon.ca/Loving-Someone-Who-Has-Dementia/dp/1118002296/ref=pd_sim_14_3?_encoding=UTF8&psc=1&refRID=2K2ZSY5G1TMVAX4APCAR*

Care and Compliance Group. "Fire Safety and Emergency Measures Preparedness" https://www.careandcompliance.com/fire-safety-and-emergency-preparedness.html

CareGiverStress.com. "Tolls of Caregiving Widespread Study Says" http://www.caregiverstress.com/stress-management/signs-of-stress/toll-of-caregiving-widespread/

Denholm, D. (2012) *The Caregiving Wife's Handbook. https://www.amazon.ca/Caregiving-Wifes-Handbook-Seriously-Yourself/dp/0897936051/ref=pd_cp_14_1?_encoding=UTF8&psc=1&refRID=15GBKEFNW8Y*

Family Caregiver Alliance. "Caregiving at Home: A Guide to Community Resources" https://www.caregiver.org/caregiving-home-guide-community-resources

Government of Canada. "Caregiver Conversations: It's about You and the Person You Support" https://www.canada.ca/en/employment-social-development/corporate/seniors/forum/care-conversation.html

Government of Canada. "Understand how Caregiving Can Affect You" https://www.canada.ca/en/employment-social-development/corporate/seniors/forum/care-conversation.html#h2.4

Jacobs, B. (2006). *The Emotional Survival Guide for Caregivers. https://www.amazon.ca/Emotional-Survival-Guide-Caregivers-Yourself/dp/1572307293/ref=pd_sbs_14_4?_encoding=UTF8&psc=1&refRID=DPBQGHCJA6GXX9R7AD2Y*

Jacobs, B. and Mayer, J. (2016) *Meditations for Caregivers. https://www.amazon.ca/AARP-Meditations-Caregivers-Practical-Emotional/dp/0738219029/ref=pd_rhf_dp_s_cp_2?_encoding=UTF8&pd_rd_i=0738219029&pd_rd_r=H2QP1C4BMYG11APXND10&pd_rd_w=p0Wx0&pd_rd_wg=vLrHH&psc=1&refRID=H2QP1C4BMYG11APXND10*

Lebow, G. (1999) *Coping with Your Difficult Older Parent. https://www.amazon.ca/Coping-Your-Difficult-Older-Parent/dp/038079750X/ref=pd_sim_14_4?_encoding=UTF8&psc=1&refRID=XG563QA85WT3CVQA1FZF*

Lynn, D. (2010). *When the Man You Love is Ill. https://www.amazon.ca/When-Man-You-Love-Ill/dp/1569242852/ref=pd_sim_14_4?_encoding=UTF8&psc=1&refRID=HKDH27EHFBPHP5RY95G4*

Mace, N. *The 36-Hour Day: A Family Guide to Dealing with People who have Alzheimer's Disease, Dementia and Related Memory Loss. https://www.amazon.ca/36-Hour-Day-Alzheimer-Disease-Dementias/dp/1455521159*

mmLearning.org. "Staying Independent Longer" training video. http://training.mmlearn.org/video-library/staying-independent-longer-with-adaptive-equipment-and-strengthening-exercises

mmLearning.org. "How to Transfer Someone from a Wheelchair to a Car" http://training.mmlearn.org/video-library/how-to-transfer-someone-from-a-wheelchair-to-a-car

mmLearning.org. "Fear of Falling Causes Falls" learning video. http://training.mmlearn.org/video-library/fear-of-falling-causes-falls
mmLearning.org. "Cultural Sensitivity" training video. http://training.mmlearn.org/video-library/question-and-answer-session

mmLearning.org. "Depression and Elderly" training video. http://training.mmlearn.org/video-library/hidden-heroes-one-couples-caregiving-story-0

Newmark, A. and Timashenka, G. (2014) Chicken Soup for the Soul: Living with Alzheimer's & Other Dementias: 101 Stories of Caregiving, Coping, and Compassion https://www.amazon.ca/Chicken-Soup-Soul-Alzheimers-Caregiving/dp/1611599342/ref=pd_lpo_sbs_14_t_2?_encoding=UTF8&psc=1&refRID=XG563QA85WT3CVQA1FZF

OSHA. "Guidelines for Prevention of Workplace Violence for Healthcare and Social Service Workers". https://www.osha.gov/Publications/osha3148.pdf

Public Health Agency of Canada. "Self-Care for Caregivers" http://www.phac-aspc.gc.ca/publicat/oes-bsu-02/caregvr-eng.php

WebMD.com "What Caregivers Should Know about Medicare". http://www.webmd.com/health-insurance/support-for-the-medicare-caregiver#1

Yancy, L. Orange County Catholic. "Six Strategies to Help Seniors Maintain Their Independence" http://occatholic.com/six-strategies-to-help-seniors-maintain-their-independence/

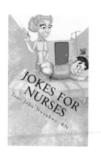 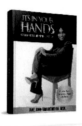 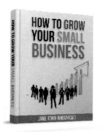 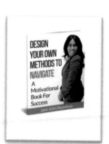 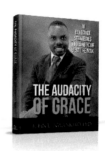

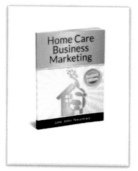 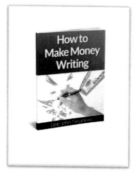 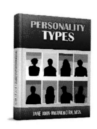 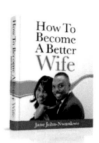

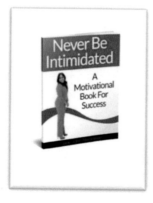 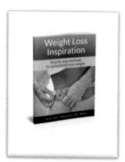 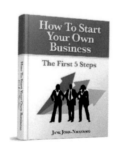 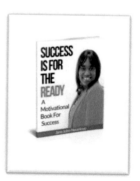

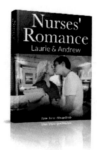 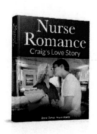 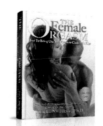 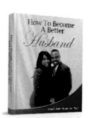

www.janejohn-nwankwo.com   Search books on Amazon.com

ABOUT THE AUTHOR

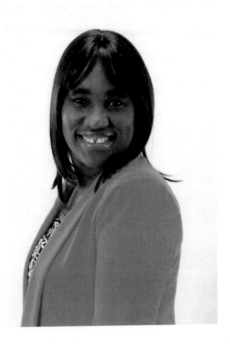

Jane John-Nwankwo CPT, RN, MSN, PHN is a motivational speaker and published author of more than 50 books which include textbooks for healthcare training, fiction for entertainment, and motivational books.

Simply search

"Books by Jane John-Nwankwo"

On Amazon.com

Visit her website:

www.janejohn-nwankwo.com

Book Jane John-Nwankwo as your motivational speaker now at
www.JaneJohn-Nwankwo.com

With more than 10 years as a professional speaker, Jane John-Nwankwo can hold any audience sitting straight on their chairs for any length of time! She is a seminar leader and a published author of more than 50 books including textbooks for healthcare training, fiction for entertainment, books for new entrepreneurs and motivational and inspirational books like the "It's in your hands" series.

She earned her Masters of Science in Nursing from University of Phoenix. She is currently an educational consultant, as well as an entrepreneurial consultant. Her speaking interests include: Motivational speeches for new business owners, Motivational speeches for any category of people, Employee seminars, Students' Empowerment, Healthcare topics, Topics related to women and any Christian topic. Book a speaking appointment today Wow! your audience. Electrify your seminar!!

www.janejohn-nwankwo.com

Having

compassion for the

elderly is a good way

to prepare for one's

own aging

-Jane John-Nwankwo

Made in the USA
Middletown, DE
21 January 2021

31620305R00100